EAT better,
FEEL better

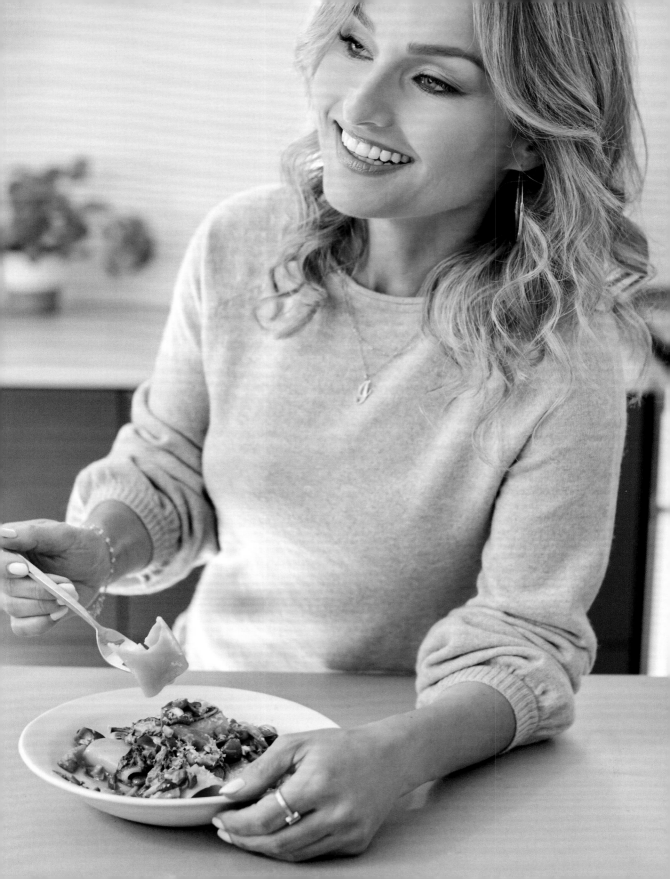

EAT
better,
FEEL
better

MY RECIPES
FOR WELLNESS AND HEALING,
INSIDE AND OUT

GIADA DE LAURENTIIS

RODALE

NEW YORK

The material in this book is for informational purposes only and is not intended as a substitute for the advice and care of your physician. The nutrition and wellness program described in this book should be followed only after first consulting with your physician to make sure it is appropriate for your individual circumstances. Keep in mind that nutritional needs vary from person to person, depending on age, sex, health status, and total diet. The author and the publisher disclaim responsibility for any adverse effects that may result from the use or application of the information contained in this book.

Published in the United States by Rodale Books, an imprint of Random House, a division of Penguin Random House LLC, New York.
rodalebooks.com

RODALE and the Plant colophon are registered trademarks of Penguin Random House LLC.

Library of Congress Cataloging-in-Publication Data has been applied for.

ISBN 978-0-593-13843-4
Ebook ISBN 978-0-593-13844-1

Printed in China

Photographs: Kristin Teig
Food styling: Lish Steiling
Food assistant: Marie Rosecleer
Prop styling: Kate Parisian
Photo assistant: David Peng

Editor: Raquel Pelzel
Book design: Mia Johnson
Production manager: Kim Tyner
Production editor: Joyce Wong
Composition: Merri Ann Morrell
Indexer: Elizabeth Parson

10 9 8 7 6 5 4 3 2 1

First Edition

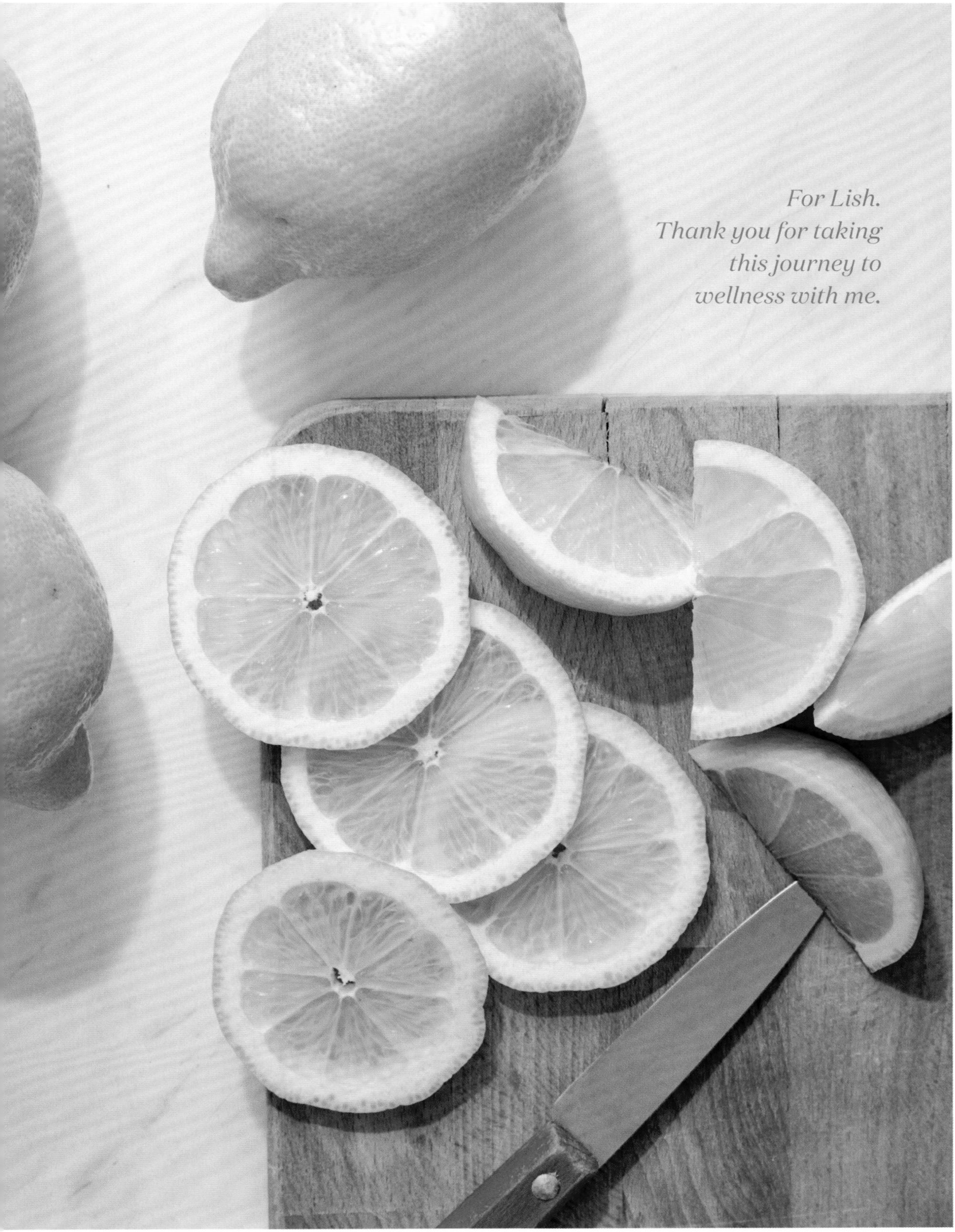

For Lish.
Thank you for taking this journey to wellness with me.

Contents

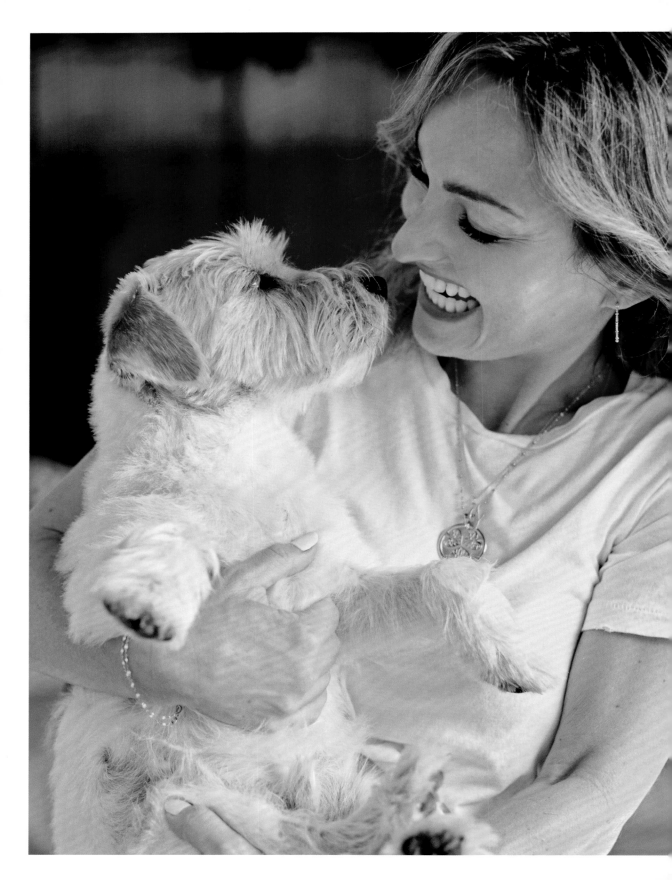

INTRODUCTION

This book is the culmination of a ten-year journey, an exploration that not so coincidentally took place between my fortieth and fiftieth birthdays. Over the last decade I've made a conscious effort to take control of my health because it had finally become impossible to ignore the fact that the choices (or lack thereof) I'd been making for the past twenty years just weren't working for me anymore.

A lot of factors brought me to this point. My forties were an incredible career-building period: I opened three restaurants and launched a website and e-commerce business, all while shooting multiple cooking shows in LA, NYC, and Italy *and* raising a daughter as a single mom. It seemed the harder I worked, the more opportunities I was offered, and I didn't want to let any of them slip away. But each new obligation meant I was spread a little thinner—always on a plane, in a car, grabbing what food and rest I could when I could. I was chronically sleep deprived, and a couple of minutes on a hotel treadmill were as close as I came to an exercise routine. Some days I barely ate enough to keep me going. I was finally attaining the kind of success I'd never even dreamed of, but a lot of the time I was too depleted to enjoy it.

And let's not forget, as a woman, knocking on the door of fifty brings its own special challenges. Along with the wisdom of experience and a newfound confidence come the joys of a slower metabolism, hormonal fluctuations, and

it's not easy to change the way you think about food, but I'm better for it every day

---

a host of physical changes, from loss of muscle mass to deepening crows' feet and wrinkles. And it's not only those of us who spend many of our days with a camera pointed in our direction who struggle with these changes; everyone wants to look and feel their best.

Tricks that had always helped me cope under pressure and compensate for too much travel, interrupted sleep, irregular and sometimes unhealthy meals—usually sugar in some form—now just made me feel *more* exhausted. Stress was omnipresent. My digestion became so sluggish and unpredictable that some days I could barely function. On top of that, my immunity was shot; I found myself getting sick constantly, and I couldn't bounce back the way I did when I was younger. I just felt like I had nothing left in the tank. I realized that if I didn't prioritize my health above the hundred other things vying for my attention, I would only continue to feel worse, not better.

So, I made changes to the way I eat—big ones. I learned to really listen to my gut and, more importantly, to respect what it was telling me instead of ignoring it or trying to figure out a workaround that would let me eat the way I always had. I came up with a program that gave my digestive system a chance to recover and heal (more on that on page 57), and an approach to eating that let my body work a little less hard at processing what I ate so it could spend more of its resources on keeping me healthy and active.

I'm not a doctor, and I don't pretend to have all the answers, but one thing I know for sure is that I feel better today than I did at thirty-five. I wasn't far into this journey before it became crystal clear to me that it all starts with food. Once I rethought the way I ate and how my body processes the fuel I feed it, it was easier to fit restorative practices like meditation, consistent exercise, and better sleep into my life. The funny thing was, far from making my days feel even more overscheduled, these self-care efforts actually created more room and freedom in my life—because I felt good so much more of the time, I had more productive hours in a day.

None of this transformation would have been possible without true and lasting changes to what I eat and how I think about food. In this book I share the recipes and philosophy that I followed—and continue to practice—to reset my digestive health, restore my gut's ability to work at peak capacity, and keep my immune system strong. My approach minimizes foods known to cause inflammation and nurtures the delicate ecosystem of the gut rather than stressing it out with toxins and irritants. And while this is not a weight-loss plan, I wouldn't be surprised if prioritizing some of these gut-friendly foods for a few weeks—or longer, if you like the way they make you feel—results in a corresponding *de*-emphasis on the foods that make you feel clogged up, bogged down, and heavy (spoiler: many of them are high in fat, carbs, and calories!). If you eat well most of the time, you may also find that when you do stray (it happens to the best of us), recovery will become more intuitive and less depleting.

Most of us will live to a ripe old age these days; the question is, what quality of life will you enjoy along the way? Wherever you are on this journey, you face a crossroads every time you put dinner on the table, or choose to flip through your phone rather than do a few minutes of yoga or meditation. I'm here to be your guide, your rooting section, and your translator as you learn to listen to your gut and use that feedback to chart your own path to wellness. I'm not gonna lie; it's not easy to change the way you think about food, but I'm better for it every day, and you will be too. In the chapters that follow you'll find a wealth of flavorful and uncomplicated recipes that will help reset your gut, twenty-one days of meal plans to help you make eating smarter a habit rather than a "diet," and all the lessons I've learned about what makes me feel stronger, healthier, and well fed, in both senses of the word.

Buon appetito—and *buona salute*!

xo

Giada

PART I

IT ALL STARTS
with FOOD

CHAPTER 1

Me and Food: Best of Frenemies

It's no accident that I ended up cooking for a living—I've always loved food. Not just eating it, although that's certainly a big part of the picture, but also the way cooking lets me express my creativity and shower the people who gather around my table with a tangible expression of my love and affection. Food has been my livelihood for three decades, and it creates a deeper connection to my family and my cultural roots. It has brought me into the lives and homes of so many people I would never have met otherwise. Plus, it's delicious! So how could I not love food?

The thing is, though, I didn't love what happened when I *ate* certain foods. Rich pastas, fried foods, ice cream, or a grilled four-cheese sandwich started to feel more like punishments than indulgences when I woke up feeling frankly lousy the next day, no matter how delicious they were. But I was so used to thinking of these foods as special treats and "comfort food" that I kept right on eating them—despite how *un*comfortable they actually made me feel.

I know I'm not the only one stuck in that unhealthy rut. You've probably noticed how certain foods affect you the next day. Imagine you have something really important to do tomorrow morning. Do you have a big plate of nachos with three-alarm salsa and chocolate ice cream for dinner? Or do you play it safe with a simple bowl of soup, or maybe some baked chicken with roasted veggies? If so, you've probably already figured out that you'll be much more present and focused if you're not dealing with bloating or cramps, or exhaustion from the acid reflux that kept you from getting a good night's sleep. Maybe you haven't made the connection yet—and you suffer the consequences, unable to bring your best self to the table because you're too busy casing the joint for a bathroom and counting the minutes before you're outta there.

Multiply that feeling by a thousand and you'll have some idea of what I was dealing with before I redefined my relationship with food and learned to hear what my gut had been trying to tell me.

I wish I could say that constant cycle of eating and regret was a recent development for me, but the truth is I've had digestive issues my whole life, even as a child. Like a lot of kids (Italian or not), I filled up on big plates of pasta and slices of white bread slathered with my favorite chocolate hazelnut spread. Vegetables and proteins came in a distant second to my beloved carbs—and they weren't "good" complex carbs, they were processed grains that really did a number on me; I was frequently constipated and bloated to the point that my parents were forced to resort to enemas to get things moving again and ease my distress. At that point—I was just a young girl—I wasn't putting it together enough to realize that what I was eating was having a big effect on how I was feeling. And with four kids to cook for, my mother wasn't looking to tailor a special diet around my tummy troubles. She came from the school of "I'm not a short-order cook; you'll eat what I make!" I was the kid with the sensitive stomach, and we basically left it at that.

My diet improved and grew more varied as I got older, no doubt due at least in some part to my family's move to Los Angeles,

where veggies and healthy food reign supreme. But that was hardly the end of my gastric woes. To the contrary, they became even more disabling when I decided to pursue a career in food. In culinary school and later, working in restaurants around Los Angeles, eating a bite of everything that came my way was practically in the job description. I was feasting on the pastries and cakes I was creating, experimenting with a new cuisine every day for my private catering clients, and maintaining a brutal schedule that kept me on my feet fifteen hours straight for days on end. I knew a lot of foods were going to be a punch in the gut for me, so my solution was to eat less, figuring I could catch up on my days off. I've never been what you would call big, but during this period I became almost alarmingly thin. And I often felt sick and tired, to the point that much of my downtime was spent recuperating in bed.

When Food Network came knocking in 2003, I was excited to be able to share my love of food with a wider audience, but that took a toll. Not to burst anyone's bubble, but filming twenty-six episodes of an instructional cooking show twice each year is a whole lot harder than it looks. My shoot days often started before dawn with hair and makeup and lasted well into the twilight hours. And all that gorgeous food I was making for the camera? That was usually scarfed up by the crew as I huddled with producers mapping out the next segment, sipping one of my ever-present Americanos. On camera, though, I couldn't control myself, especially around the sweet stuff. If they wanted to shoot me taking a bite of a brownie or cookie, I was like, "No problem, how many takes do you need?"

The stress of my production schedule was compounded as I layered on the new responsibilities of writing cookbooks, managing retail partnerships, and maintaining a full schedule of appearances—not to mention my obligations to my family and husband. I don't regret a minute of it, and all of these opportunities gave me a chance to learn and grow and succeed in a million different ways, but it was just nonstop. To keep up my energy when all I really felt like doing was crawling into bed for the world's longest nap, I relied on my two favorite energy boosters: caffeine and sugar. And I'm not talking about those chaste little squares of 78% cacao dark chocolate everyone talks about; I went hard on cookies, sugary muffins, or fistfuls of chocolate chips that I'd swipe off the set. If I couldn't get my hands on anything else, I would even dip sugar cubes into my coffee and crunch them down whole or dump multiple packets of sugar into an iced tea and suck up the sodden sugar with a straw.

Once those sugar-fueled energy spikes had run their course, though, I found myself more exhausted than ever, usually too beat to even contemplate making a real dinner. Too many nights I resorted to ordering in or dining out, always tempted by a rich, cheesy pasta I might want to feature on my show plus, of course, a decadent dessert

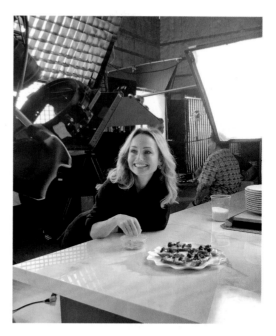

On my set in Los Angeles.

to top it all off! Even worse were the travel days, when my main source of sustenance was whatever I could grab at the airport or something off the late-night room service menu. Fries and ice cream, or chocolate espresso beans from the minibar at midnight? I told myself it was better than nothing, although deep down I knew better.

The effects of this endless cycle of spike-and-crash eating were brutal. Bloating, frequent stomach pains, gas, and acid reflux were everyday events. Some days I simply felt overwhelmed, but I just chalked it up to being overworked. I was foggy, irritable, tired, and weak, and I didn't have the resilience to fight off even

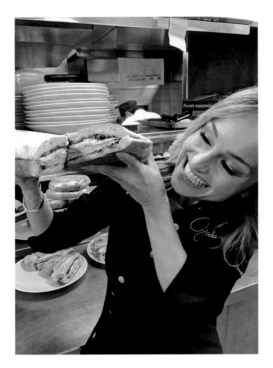

In my kitchen at Giada in Las Vegas.

comfortable on my not-so-big frame was never really my problem, and to a large extent I can thank genetics for that (if you've ever seen a photo of my gorgeous seventy-year-old mother, Veronica, you know I come by it naturally). Instead, my unhealthy eating was taking a toll on me in ways that were less visible to the outside world. I had chronic rosacea and edema (swelling) under my eyes. Near-constant constipation and bloating were starting to limit the way I moved through life. Every cold turned into a sinus infection or bronchitis. In hindsight, the cause of all these symptoms should have been obvious, but somehow I convinced myself that someone who knew as much about food as I did couldn't be brought down by her diet. Instead, I kept going to different doctors looking for a silver bullet.

It was also around this time that my marriage of twenty years broke down, leaving me with a five-year-old daughter to care for, and all the financial and emotional fallout that comes with ending a significant relationship. As these things go, our divorce was relatively civil, but even the best divorce is a wrenching experience and a major contributor to day-to-day stress. My first restaurant had just opened, too, and that learning curve was steep. It was just . . . a lot.

The final straw was a case of sinusitis that I couldn't shake for months. I went to the doctor time and again, only to be sent home with another prescription for antibiotics. But it never completely went away, and every time I got on a plane it

the mildest of colds that might be going around. When I did get sick, it took me longer than it should have to recover; a three-day chill-out wasn't enough to get me back on track the way it had been when I was in my twenties.

Through it all, people were *always* asking what my secret was for remaining slim while dishing up all that incredible pasta, and pizza, and risotto. I always smiled and responded, "I eat a little of everything . . . just not a lot of anything!" But portion control wasn't the whole truth. To be honest, maintaining a weight that is seemed I emerged at my destination with a full-blown infection, complete with body aches, fever, and the kind of fatigue not even a triple shot of espresso could overcome. It got to the point that I was taking antibiotics every day as a precaution, which wreaked such havoc on my whole digestive system that I woke up every morning wondering if I'd be able to make that 6:00 a.m. call time at the *Today* show or spend eight hours on a photo set without anyone realizing how fragile I was.

I knew something had to give, and I also knew that the doctors I'd been seeing didn't have the answers I needed. I began working with Dr. Deborah Kim, an acupuncturist, nutritionist, and master herbalist who is well versed in Eastern medicine, hoping that she could relieve my sinus issues. It was she who first suggested I needed to think seriously about the way I was eating. Under her guidance I went on a regimen of superclean, ultrarestrictive meals for about a week, and to my amazement, I felt better almost immediately. As the bloat diminished and my sluggish digestion improved, I found I had more pep in my step. The fog in my brain began to clear. It was like the sun had finally come out.

It seems crazy that no one had ever suggested I make changes to my diet—or maybe they had, but I just wasn't ready to hear them. You know how we tend to block out the things we really don't want to deal with. But after feeling the undeniable benefits of that week-long cleanse, the inspiration for my three-day reboot plan on

page 57, I knew food and I needed to fix our busted relationship. I was finally ready.

Working with Dr. Kim's recommendations, coupled with my own suspicions about which foods I really didn't handle well, I began to reprioritize what I was eating. Foods like dairy, certain legumes, and refined wheat that were hard to digest and made my gut work overtime went to the back of the line; those that were easy on my stomach and provided abundant quantities of the clean nutrients I needed, foods like greens, vegetables, and sweet potatoes supplemented by a little bit of lean protein, went front and center. Once I saw how sugar, alcohol, and animal fats had been taxing my gut, liver, and kidneys, creating a hostile environment for good digestive microbes and causing inflammation, it became much easier to eat less of them. I also eliminated toxins by cutting back on certain types of fish, commercially produced meat, and packaged foods. Now, when I eat animal products, I try to make sure they are as clean as possible, meaning free-range and/or grass-fed, free of hormones, pesticides, and other chemical contaminants whenever possible.

Dr. Kim also taught me that even when we eat a "healthy diet," we are not necessarily getting all the nutrients we need. Let's face it, food production has changed a lot over the past fifty years; modern farming practices that favor appearance and transportability over nutrition, the extensive use of chemical fertilizers and drugs on livestock, and a decrease in the diversity of the varieties and strains of foods have all compromised the nutritional value of what is on our tables. Even if we were to eat exactly like our great-grandparents did—and most of us don't—we wouldn't get the same benefits they did, because most modern foods simply don't have the same nutritional profile as they might have even fifty years ago. To put it plainly, many of the foods we eat today have had the goodness bred or processed out of them.

I began to approach cooking and eating by thinking about micronutrients—vitamins, essential fatty acids, and antioxidants—rather than just focusing on carbs, fats, and proteins, also known as macronutrients. After all, both salmon and greens on a bed of quinoa and a burger deluxe with fries can be defined as a serving of protein, carbs, and fat, but one is delivering a lot more food value than the other, value that can't really be tallied if you look only at the macronutrient picture.

Look, most of us make an effort to eat well. I know I thought I did! But along with the kale salads and grilled skinless chicken breasts, we are all consuming too many foods that simply aren't doing us any good. Worse, they may be slowing us down, causing an inflammatory effect in our guts, compromising our immunity, and keeping us from living our best lives. A food that's supposedly a "treat" is a lot less tempting if it results in an unhappy gut with all that that implies. I eventually realized that those "cheat" meals were actually cheating me out of whole days as my digestion struggled to process them.

Once I understood that, the choice became simple: I had to think before I ate. Now foods that are nutritionally dense, that are free of contaminants and environmental toxins, and that don't put a strain on my immune system are the backbone of my diet. Anything that doesn't reach that high bar, or that I *know* will make me feel lousy the next day, like heavy fried foods, sugary treats, and rich cream sauces, goes into the category of "proceed with caution." It's not that I never eat these foods, but now that I understand how they affect me, most of the time (well, at least a lot of the time) I choose feeling good over the momentary pleasure of a chocolate chip cookie.

It's not a radical change. As you'll see when you get to the recipe section starting on page 76, my cooking still reflects the amazing ingredients and flavors of the Italian cuisine that I love best. I've just tweaked it a bit to make me feel and function my best.

Eating better and making more conscious choices about how, what, and why I eat is just one of the ways I'm learning to take control of my health. In chapter 7, I'll also share some of the lifestyle changes I've made to mitigate the toll that things like stress and aging take on my body, no matter how virtuous I am! But it all starts with the food, and it's my goal to make this transition as easy—and delicious—as I can.

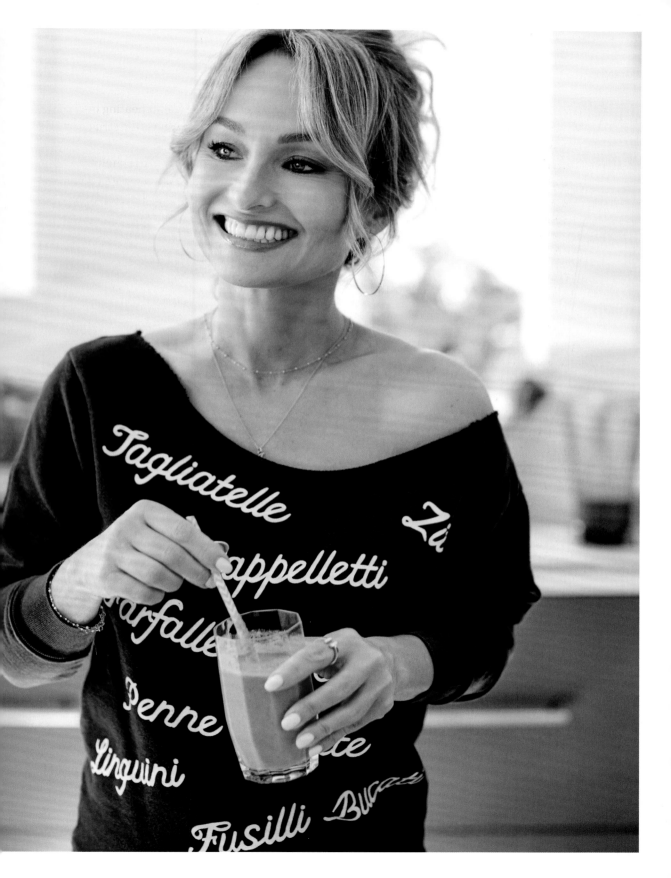

CHAPTER 2

Learning to Listen to Your Gut

I recently spent an afternoon with a group of young women who had gathered for a baby shower. The hostess had provided a spread of Southern favorites, and as the guests loaded their plates with cornbread, chicken and waffles, and mac 'n' cheese, I saw more than one roll her eyes, saying, "I'm gonna pay for *this* tonight." Turns out that nearly half of these women, all in their twenties and thirties, had serious gastrointestinal conditions and routinely popped medication to address digestive troubles.

As we chatted, I learned that many of them coped with these problems by restricting their diets to an unbelievable degree, subsisting on pasta and packaged salad mixes whenever they "cooked" at home because it seemed healthy. More than one said she never kept anything sweet or highly caloric in the house, because she

or her partner could eat an entire box of cereal before bed or demolish half a leftover pizza or jar of peanut butter if left to their own devices. The only way to control that kind of binge eating was to keep their cupboards practically bare. And when you go out, I asked, what do you eat then? "Oh, those are 'sex before dinner' nights," one of them told me with a laugh. "That way I can eat what I want, and it doesn't matter if I end up in the bathroom all night!" Super romantic, right? How did this become the new normal?

Even in "healthy" LA, where I live, too many people are trying to drown out the messages from their stressed-out guts by medicating away the symptoms with antacids, dealing with the aftermath, or giving up altogether and eating in a way that doesn't come close to providing the variety of foods and nutrients our bodies need to function well. And they're not alone; nationwide, more cases of IBS, Crohn's, GERD, and plain old heartburn and gas are being treated than ever before.

These distress signals from your gut are about more than just a tummy ache or a mad dash to the bathroom. As I've learned from experience, the effects of a disrupted digestive system can reverberate throughout your body, causing fatigue, aches and pains, skin issues, an over- or underactive immune system, and, ultimately, serious disease.

You've probably heard scientists or nutritionists refer to the microbiome, another name for the ecosystem of hardworking bacteria that inhabit your digestive system. When that ecosystem is balanced and healthy, those bacteria break down the food you eat to make its nutrients available to your organs, and to keep things moving smoothly so that toxins and by-products can be eliminated from your body. When the friendly bacteria are too busy trying to fix damage done to your gut by inflammatory foods, or get crowded out by hostile, less benign bacteria—that's when you start to feel the effects of a system that isn't working like it should. The good guys are so busy putting out fires, they can't do their day jobs of keeping your immune system strong and your body healthy.

The question is, once those friendly bacteria—aka your gut flora—send up a flare letting you know they are on the ropes, what do you do with that information? Are you going to medicate the symptoms (IBS, constipation, heartburn, and the like) into submission? Or are you ready to get at the source of all that discomfort?

BRING YOUR DOCTOR INTO THE CONVERSATION

It's essential to underscore here that *no diet, no matter how healthy*, is a substitute for routine medical care. Whenever I've made significant changes to my diet, I've done so in consultation with my doctors. My doctors also monitor my liver, kidney, and thyroid functions and do blood tests to ensure that I'm getting the essential nutrients I need—and that my levels of toxins, such as mercury, are within the normal range. If you have severe digestive problems, including stomach pains, sudden weight gain or loss, or constant diarrhea, these may indicate serious conditions that require a doctor's care and medication. Do yourself a favor and get checked out regularly.

WHAT IS INFLAMMATION, ANYWAY?

Though they sound similar, heartburn and related problems like acid reflux are not exactly the same as inflammation in the digestive system. Reflux and the like can result when the pH balance in your stomach becomes too acidic, which can cause an actual burning sensation as the acid escapes the stomach and heads up toward your esophagus. Inflammation, on the other hand, occurs when the body's immune system gets the signal to swarm something it thinks is attacking your gut. That something can be a toxin, a nasty microbe, or a protein it can't break down, like those in gluten or dairy. When your body has to deal with those perceived enemies too often, the inflammation can become chronic and spread throughout the body. In the most serious cases the immune response can go into overdrive, causing your body to attack even healthy cells, resulting in a ripple effect of problems, from fatigue to pain to a host of autoimmune diseases. Fortunately, in the case of both gut inflammation and reflux or garden-variety heartburn, eating cleaner and smarter is the first step toward putting out the fire, and there is a good deal of overlap in foods that cause one or both of these.

For me, changing what I ate and the way I thought about food has made the difference between always feeling a little bit off (or downright sick) and feeling strong, energetic, and resilient most of the time. There is a lot of talk about genes being our destiny, and I believe that genetic predispositions are a real thing. (I'm definitely not the only one in my family who suffers from digestive problems!) But the way you play your cards will ultimately have a bigger impact on how you feel than the hand you were dealt at birth. Lifestyle—diet, sleep, exercise—can actually change those biomarkers. Put simply, the choices you make about what goes into your mouth will make a *huge* difference in how you feel—not just today, but over the whole course of your life.

This is how one of my doctors explained it to me: when we eat, the toxins and inflammatory foods we put into our body go into a virtual "bucket"; when that bucket gets full to the brim and overflows, it sends our body into the black zone, which is sickness. I'm talking about scary stuff: cancer, autoimmune disease, diabetes, and gastrointestinal issues. I truly believe that the lifestyle changes I have made, especially reevaluating the way I eat, have kept *my* bucket in the gray zone. It's not empty—not by a long shot—but I don't have to worry that a slice of pizza or a bite of a doughnut is going to make it slosh over.

Identifying which foods really put your gut through the wringer is the first step, and everyone's list is going to be a little bit different. I have friends who can eat a raw kale salad every single day, but raw kale is a now-and-then thing for me. On the other hand, I can eat a mountain of bitter broccoli rabe or a big radicchio salad without batting an eyelash. Some grains agree with me more than others, and cauliflower, everyone's new best friend, makes me crazy bloated. Go figure.

For me, keeping toxins and specific foods that cause inflammation out of my system has become the priority. I'm what doctors call a low detoxifier. That means it takes longer for my liver, gallbladder, and other organs to process out harmful factors. The result is that toxins tend to accumulate in my body, causing—you guessed it— inflammation. I also find that I need to watch acidic foods like caffeine, citrus juices, and alcohol, as well as other things that cause the production of too much stomach acid, like rich, super spicy, or fried foods.

Proceed with Caution

You probably already have some idea of which foods are a little harder for your stomach to handle. You may even have been tested for intolerance or sensitivities to things like dairy or gluten. But even if you don't know for sure which foods give you trouble, the following list is a good place to start. It includes food categories that are generally acknowledged to make the digestion work overtime and promote an unhealthy environment in the gut that can, in turn, lead to problems throughout the body. It also includes foods that may not by themselves be harmful, but are too often handled in a way that makes them less than healthy by the time they get to you, whether that means they've been raised with hormones and pesticides, or had all their goodness compromised by additives or processing. These are the biggies:

1. Sugar: I could have made this numbers 1, 2, and 3—that's how much I struggle with sugar. Until I made a real effort to tamp down how much sugar I ate, for me it wasn't a treat, it was a legitimate addiction, the ultimate bad boyfriend, luring me back time and again even though I knew I'd hate myself in the morning. Really, the only good thing I can say about sugar is that the less you eat of it, the less you crave it, but breaking that habit has been *hard,* and it's an ongoing battle. That said, it's one worth fighting. A ton has been written about the effects of sugar on our health, particularly the refined sugar in sweet things like desserts, candy, and soda, which

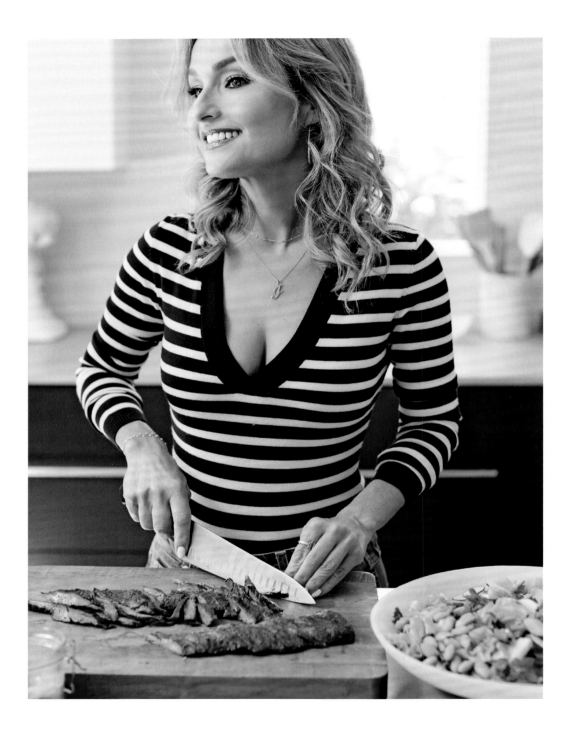

has been shown to cause inflammation, spike blood sugar, and affect the body's ability to make or use the insulin needed to convert sugars to energy. Another knock against sugar is the company it keeps; when you munch on something sweet, you're probably also consuming a bunch of refined grains, bad fats, or dairy, any one of which could be foods that trigger an inflammatory response in your gut. These days there is sugar lurking in nearly everything that comes in a package, from jarred spaghetti sauce to your morning yogurt, so check labels and skip the packaged food (see #9) whenever you can.

2. Dairy: For many people, dairy is inflammatory because it contains sugars in the form of lactose, and if you don't produce the enzymes necessary to break down those sugars, it can result in bloating, gas, and related gastric problems. Even if you are able to process lactose, you may be sensitive to the proteins in dairy, resulting in—once again—stomach woes. Moreover, the majority of the dairy products we buy come from animals that have been treated with hormones and antibiotics, and they often contain a fair amount of unhealthy animal fats. The proteins in dairy products made from sheep's and goat's milk differ somewhat from those in cow's milk, and for that reason some people find them easier to digest. If dairy is one of your big problems, try switching to goat cheese or sheep's milk yogurt or a nondairy alternative (try my recipe for dairy-free almond milk on

page 104) and see if your body likes them better. For this book I haven't eliminated dairy entirely—you'll never get me to give up my Parmigiano-Reggiano! That said, if I can use dairy more sparingly without compromising the flavor of a recipe, I do.

3. Red meat: I'm not anti–red meat—I like a good Bolognese or even a steak now and then—but I'm not a big fan of how a lot of the meat we eat is produced. Too often they are raised in inhumane, crowded conditions, given pesticide-laden feed their systems were not designed to digest, and routinely dosed with hormones and antibiotics to counter the effects of their poor living conditions. Pasture-raised animals are one solution, but this is an expensive option that isn't readily available to everyone.

That said, the nutrients we get from meat, especially B vitamins, are hard to get from other foods, so I do eat red meat now and then. However, I think of it as the side dish, not the main event, and keep servings to a palm-size portion (that's about 4 ounces for me). If I eat more than that, I find it sits in my stomach and makes me feel heavy, weighted down, and bloated. I often incorporate lamb into my menus because it's not mass produced in the same way beef and pork are, and it satisfies my taste for red meat. Speaking of pork, I choose a heritage breed, like Berkshire, when possible, and eat highly processed and preserved products, like salami, bacon, and even pancetta, only occasionally.

4. Refined grains and carbs: I'm not the first to talk about the virtues of whole grains over their pulverized, sanitized, nutrient-stripped counterparts, and I won't be the last: it's hard to overstate how differently your gut reacts to a serving of whole-grain farro or quinoa than it does to a slice of white bread. One gives the microbes that live in your gut the stuff they like to eat—probiotic fiber—and all the antioxidants and micronutrients found in the bran and kernel of the grain, so it goes through your system more slowly and provides sustained energy. The refined carbs in that white bread, on the other hand, barge right through the express lane, causing inflammation without providing much in the way of nutrition. Which brings us to . . .

5. Gluten: There's been plenty of debate about the extent and severity of gluten sensitivities in the general population, and how sensitivity differs from a true intolerance, as in the case of celiac disease. Fortunately, these severe intolerances are relatively rare, but it does seem clear that the proteins in modern wheat and other gluten-containing grains like rye can cause inflammation in many people. Gluten also lurks in many processed foods, including soy sauce. Celiac can be identified with a blood test, so if you are concerned, ask your doctor if you should be checked out. But regardless, gluten nearly always goes hand in hand with high-carb processed foods, like white bread, pizza, and baked goods

or pastas made from highly refined wheat flour—things that you should be sidelining anyway if you are eating with gut health in mind.

FRY-BY-NIGHT FOODS

Proceed with Caution is really more a cooking method than a particular food category, but if you want to do your body some good, say no thanks next time you're asked, "Do you want fries with that?" I'm not saying all fat is evil—that's just not true. Fat provides essential fatty acids and helps us absorb certain nutrients, a key to good health. Fat is also satisfying; it gives food richness, it carries flavor, and it helps us feel full longer—all good qualities. And our brains need fat to work! But when some fats are exposed to high heat, they change chemically, becoming much harder for your body to break down. These so-called trans fats are associated with serious health concerns. (Plus, like all fats, trans fats are highly caloric, but without the heart-healthy benefits that come with unsaturated fats.) You will get the same stomach-filling effect from avocados and olive oil, fatty fish, and lean meats with far less downside than you will from fries and chips.

6. Caffeine: Medical science has been going back and forth on this one for years, with some studies showing it to be harmful and others suggesting it is actually beneficial in fighting cancer and other diseases. The one thing we know for sure, though, is that it will keep you from getting the sleep you need, particularly if you drink it close to bedtime, as its effects can last for hours. For that reason, I limit the amount of caffeine I drink—and that includes black and green teas—and avoid it altogether after noon.

7. Alcohol: When it comes to alcohol, moderation is key. Alcohol is known to put a strain on your liver and cause inflammation. Overconsumption of alcohol has also been shown to disrupt sleep, preventing you from getting the deep, sustained rest you need. Because I'm one of those folks whose liver is a slow detoxifier, I limit my drinking to one or two glasses of wine per week, and I avoid sugary, fruity drinks or wines with additives like sulfites.

8. Nightshades: This group of fruits and vegetables includes eggplants, tomatoes, peppers, and potatoes (although not sweet potatoes, which are not related to their white counterparts botanically). All of these foods contain alkaloids, which have been shown to cause inflammation; this is why some people, especially those with serious autoimmune diseases, choose to avoid them. The medical community is not unanimous in supporting this theory,

but there does seem to be consensus that if someone is already fighting inflammatory symptoms, eating these foods can exacerbate the situation. You're never going to get an Italian cook to give up tomatoes entirely (or my beloved Calabrian chile paste!), but I use them with more restraint these days, and you may want to as well, especially when you aren't feeling great.

9. Processed foods: By this I mean anything that comes in a box, can, or jar. When foods go through the process of being refined, combined, and packaged, you are always going to lose something in translation—usually nutrients, or good stuff like fiber—and in return, pick up things that you don't want, like chemical preservatives, stabilizers, and added sugars, salt, and fat. Even things that seem completely natural and unadulterated are usually treated with preservatives to prolong their shelf life. Check out the label of that shredded cheese you bought to save a few minutes when making dinner. I bet it contains anticaking agents, like cornstarch or potato starch, and some kind of mold retardant. And if shredded cheese has that much baggage, just imagine what's in that bottle of barbecue sauce or frozen pizza! Do you really want to be eating all those additives?

I'm not going to pretend that I don't take shortcuts in the kitchen now and then, and a lot of these convenience foods make life a little easier. After all, there are only so many hours in the day, and any time you cook a meal at home rather than order in (or do drive-through), it's a win. But these days I'm all about eating intentionally. If I'm going to eat something that contains sugar or gluten or another not-the-best ingredient, I want to do so consciously, not just let unwanted chemicals and additives piggyback their way into my gut for the sake of saving a few minutes of grating cheese or making my own salad dressing. Using as few things as possible that come out of a package simply helps me better control what I'm eating.

All the recipes in this book make minimal use of Proceed with Caution, and even if you don't think you have a problem processing certain foods, you'll never know how much better you might feel without them if you don't give it a try (see page 49 for my meal plans if you want to see what eating really clean looks like week by week). If, after forgoing one of the naughties for a stretch, you want to reintroduce it, go ahead. Just note any changes in your digestion, energy levels, moods, or how your skin looks. I bet you'll be surprised to find that foods you thought you tolerated just fine actually cause more problems than you realized. Better still, you may be shocked to see how little you miss them when you use my recipes.

The bottom line is that we all react to foods differently, and these reactions can also change over time; sometimes foods we could eat without a second thought when we

NEVER SAY NEVER

Time out for an important note: Unless you have a true intolerance or diagnosed disease like celiac, eating well is *not* about eliminating foods; it's about noting how they affect you and eating *less* of those that challenge your health. Pasta is not the enemy and neither is dairy, and no Italian chef would ever tell you otherwise. Eating well is about finding the right balance for *you*. As I've gotten older, I find cutting out foods I crave affects me more than it used to, not less, and if you think for one second I wouldn't be dreaming all day long about things I've denied myself, you are wrong.

Sometimes it's just better to give in to the cravings in a moderate, controlled way. I wish I could say I'm the kind of person who can eat a spoonful of frozen berries when I'm dying for chocolate, but that's simply not true. Instead, a square of the real thing, stored in the fridge so that it melts slowly in my mouth, quells that craving better than a heaping helping of a less satisfying replacement.

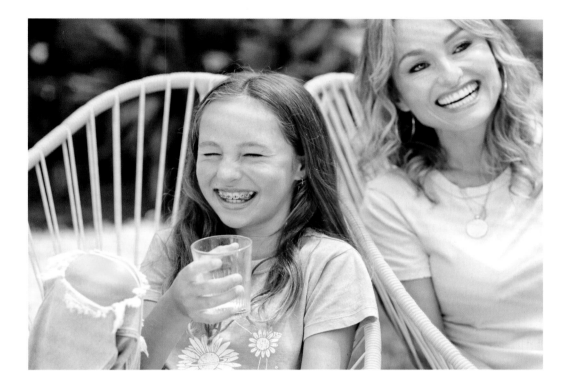

were younger now bring us right to the brink of the danger zone because the stomach lining thins with age, and our ability to produce stomach acid decreases. By eating more nutrient-dense, anti-inflammatory foods and antioxidants (molecules that fight free radicals in your body—a cause of illness and aging—and are found in vegetables, fruits, nuts, and other foods, like dark chocolate) and eating everything else more mindfully, you are going to be that much further ahead of the game, *whatever* your personal Achilles' heel. Listen to your gut; it won't steer you wrong.

Remember, the real goal here is to reduce the amount of inflammatory foods and toxins we put in our body, not to take anything off the menu entirely. If you eat bad stuff, do so consciously. Tell yourself: Today I went overboard. Tomorrow I will do better. Beating yourself up won't make you feel better, but getting a little bit healthier and more mindful every day will. You may just decide to eat certain foods less and less often once you see how great eating this way makes you feel.

And now on to the good stuff—the gut-friendly foods I can't get enough of!

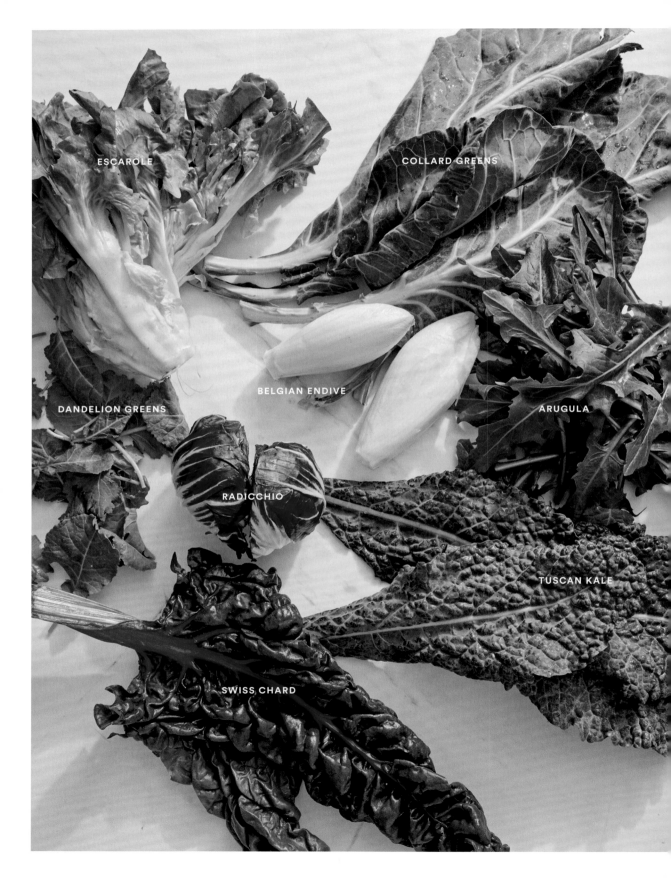

ESCAROLE

COLLARD GREENS

BELGIAN ENDIVE

DANDELION GREENS

ARUGULA

RADICCHIO

TUSCAN KALE

SWISS CHARD

CHAPTER 3

Foods That Help

The recipes in this book are designed to cut your gut some slack so it's not spending all its energy trying to digest things that *cause* inflammation instead of healing damage done in the past. The good news is that while some foods make your gut work overtime, there are just as many delicious, indulgent, soul-satisfying foods that can make your gut happy. As my nutritionist and acupuncturist Dr. Kim likes to remind me, we need to think of food as medicine. That means looking at everything you eat in terms of how it will make you feel: Is this going to support the delicate ecosystem that is your first line of defense against illness, or kick it when it's down?

Day to day, that means lots of vegetables make up the bulk of my diet, plus a little bit of lean protein (and not at every meal, or even every day), plenty of good fats (like olive oil) and other foods that are rich in antioxidants (score one for dark chocolate!), and a considered amount of whole, minimally processed grains. Foods known to cause inflammation, or to compromise digestive health (and I'll go into that in more depth in the next chapter), have been pushed to the margins. I haven't made any food truly off-limits; I just keep the things I know my body wants and needs at the center of the plate. In a way, it's not that different from how my grandparents approached food when I was growing up in Italy.

At first glance I think you'll find the food in this book looks pretty much like the recipes I've been sharing with you since I first published *Everyday Italian*: Italian favorites given a fresher, lighter spin; lots of yummy pastas; irresistible salads that are hearty enough to be a meal; and, of course, some truly decadent desserts. I've just nudged them away from foods I've found are hard on some people's systems (including my own) and toward nutrient-dense, gut-friendly foods full of bright flavors.

Fortunately, even when the shift away from certain types of foods is subtle, the effect can be profound. Better still, if you eat well most of the time, you'll have more reserves and resilience to deal with the occasional missteps, and recovery will become more intuitive and less depleting.

YOUR DAY-TO-DAY SHOPPING LIST: JUST THE BASICS

The recipes in this book don't constitute some kind of huge culinary about-face for me; as always, they are based on the touchstones every Italian cook lives by: fresh, whole foods, cooked simply and cleanly. I haven't banished anything from my kitchen, just shifted the balance away from big plates of pasta and meat-centric dinners to meals in which meat plays a secondary role and pasta (and other grains) is the backdrop to more vegetables (and less cheese!) than I've served in the past. Dairy, sugar, and the rest of the Proceed with Caution list (page 23) are things I eat judiciously and less frequently, and I make sure that when I do indulge, every delicious bite counts.

Now when I shop or plan a menu, the following twelve foods are my starting place.

The Delectable Dozen

1. Dark leafy greens: If spinach and romaine lettuce constitute the beginning and end of your leafy green spectrum, getting to know the varieties you've been missing out on is going to be a revelation. Lucky you! These are some of the healthiest, most nutritious foods you can put on your table, and the more of them you eat, the more you will come to love them.

Many—including collards, beet greens, and of course kale—can be eaten either cooked or raw (especially when young and tender). Expand your greens universe to include turnip greens, dandelion greens, red (Russian) kale, and my favorite, arugula, and try to include greens in two meals every day. It's easier than you think—just toss a handful into your morning smoothie or scatter some over your avocado toast; use raw or steamed greens as a bed for grilled meat or fish; or add a cup to any vegetable soup or grain bowl. *Eat leafy greens in virtually unlimited quantities.*

2. Cruciferous veggies: These include all those plants in the cabbage family—think broccoli and broccoli rabe, cauliflower, bok choy, Brussels sprouts, and kale—as well as radishes, turnips, and lots of greens (see above), from chard to watercress. These vegetables are nutritional powerhouses, full of vitamins and phytonutrients as well as fiber, and are known to be disease fighters. You'll find a bunch of new ways to use them throughout this book. *Eat as much as you want, whenever you want.*

3. Fish and seafood: I know many people are reluctant to prepare fish at home because they're afraid the cooking smells will linger, or they don't have a reliable fish store nearby, or they just plain don't love fish. But I can counter all those excuses with just as many reasons to put fish at the top of your shopping list! Fish can be an amazing source of clean, lean protein (and omega-3 fatty acids); it rarely takes longer than ten minutes to cook; and you can pair it with so many different flavors that there is certain to be a recipe that makes you a fish convert. I find most people do like salmon and shrimp, but why not branch out occasionally: give mildly flavored trout, sole, and cod a try. Small, oily fish like sardines, anchovies, and mackerel are especially good choices, as they are sustainable and the highest in good fatty acids, but be sure they are superfresh, as even a day too long out of the water can turn those oils "fishy" and unappealing. If convenience is a factor, consider buying frozen fillets. Much of the fish in our markets is shipped frozen anyway, and keeping frozen salmon or cod fillets in the freezer means you don't need to make a special trip; just throw them in the fridge in the morning and they'll be thawed for dinner. *Eat two or three servings per week.*

4. Lean animal proteins: Protein is one of the essential macronutrients our bodies require, and I think it is part of a healthy diet when eaten *in moderation*. That means a serving of 4 to 6 ounces of chicken, turkey, lean beef like skirt steak or tenderloin (not a 12-ounce steak!), lamb, or pork once or twice a week. I like to think of meat as the side dish rather than the main event, with one or two vegetables making up the bulk of the

NO FISHING

I love fish and, full disclosure, I am mostly pescatarian during the week. That said, I try to be conscious of how the fish I eat is raised. Mercury accumulation has been an issue for me in the past, and many of the big fish, including tuna (even the kind in cans!) and swordfish, can have high mercury levels. I also try to avoid farmed fish and shrimp, which are often treated with antibiotics and raised in conditions that are harmful to the environment, though I recognize that wild-caught seafood is usually pricier. Freshwater fish like trout are less likely to have mercury exposure, and if you are going for saltwater fish, opt for smaller fish, like salmon, flounder, Mediterranean sea bass, sardines, or mackerel, and make wild-caught choices when you can.

meal. This lets me enjoy the satisfying chew and flavor of meat, but I feel less weighed down. I am also choosy about the meat I buy, especially chicken and beef, which are more likely to be raised in factory-farm conditions and all that entails. Most markets now offer pastured, hormone- and antibiotic-free brands, and if your budget allows, they are smart choices. *Eat no more than four servings per week, only one of them red meat.*

PROBIOTICS VERSUS PREBIOTICS

You've probably heard these words thrown around a lot, and it seems like everything from yogurt to orange juice claims to contain probiotics these days. But what's the difference between the two? Here's all you really need to know: Probiotics are live, gut-friendly microbes found in foods with active cultures like yogurt, in fermented foods like sauerkraut, and of course in supplements. Prebiotics are the things those microbes (including the ones that already live in your gut) like to eat, such as the nonsoluble fiber in whole grains and most vegetables and fruits. If you eat a lot of probiotic foods but no prebiotics, it's like throwing a party and forgetting to put out any snacks; eventually the guests won't stick around (and even the hosts will get hungry!). So be sure to get plenty of both. I take a probiotic supplement every day and feed those bugs lots and lots of greens!

5. Eggs: Eggs are the ultimate comeback kid. Once vilified as a high-cholesterol enemy, they're now thought to be better protein sources than foods with high levels of saturated fat, and not a contributor to high blood cholesterol after all. That's good news, because they are a true convenience food, always there in the fridge for a quick dinner omelet, breakfast frittata, or portable hard-boiled snack. As with all animal proteins, choose the cleanest, most humanely raised option you can. *Eat up to six per week (including in baked goods).*

6. Whole grains: Nature knows what it's doing, which is why a grain in its whole, unrefined form is the complete nutritional package, full of fiber, antioxidants, and B vitamins. Refining strips away the bran and germ, where all those good nutrients reside, and leaves only the endosperm, the very unsexy name for the starchy part of the grain that is mostly carbs and is used to make white flour and white rice. I find whole grains like brown rice and quinoa a lot more satisfying than white rice or even polenta, both because the fiber is filling and also because they are nuttier and more toothsome. And if you get into making them in big batches to refrigerate or even freeze, they become really convenient to incorporate into meals on the fly. I love them! That said, I don't eat grains in unlimited quantities, because, whole or refined, they are still carbs, which the body converts into sugar to burn as fuel, and they make me feel really full for a long, long time. *Have up to 1 cup per day.*

7. Low-glycemic fruits: All fruit contains sugar (as do many vegetables for that matter). But when you eat the whole fruit (as opposed to simply drinking the juice), you are also getting plenty of fiber, which helps slow the absorption of those sugars into your bloodstream. (Once again, nature knows best.) Some fruits—berries, stone fruits, apples—don't cause your blood sugar to spike as strongly as others; these are the fruits I use most often in my recipes. *Have just one or two servings per day.*

8. Sweet potatoes and squash: I like sweet potatoes so much that sometimes I eat them as a snack right out of the oven, maybe sprinkled with a little salt or some spices. I like to play with different varieties, including nutty Japanese sweet potatoes and ones with yellow, white, or purple flesh, but I like Garnet sweets, with their dark red skins and moist flesh, best of all. They are less fibrous, which makes them perfect for baking and mashing. Both sweet potatoes and orange squash, like butternut and delicata, have tons of beta-carotene, vitamins, and fiber, making them a filling, healthy, and colorful addition to your plate—all good things! *Have no more than one serving per day.*

9. Nuts and seeds: Unsaturated fats, fiber, and heart-healthy nutrients are all great reasons to eat nuts, but I love them even more for the crunch, richness, and flavor they add to dishes. Meaty walnuts are my favorites, but I'm also a big fan of pepitas and neutral-flavored almonds, especially for baking. They do qualify as a high-calorie food, so don't go overboard, but when you're looking to give something a little extra flavor and texture, or craving a healthier snack, eat nuts. *Have up to ½ cup per day.*

GO GLUTEN-FREE OR NOT?

Among the few exceptions I make to the no-phony-foods rule are gluten-free pasta, bread, and panko. While many contain a laundry list of ingredients that I might not recommend on their own, I'd never sentence anyone to a life without pasta or French toast, and for people who cannot process gluten, these alternatives are lifesavers. Gluten-free panko fries up crisp and adds a hint of crunch to sheet pan dinners like the shrimp on page 202. But if gluten is not an issue for you, stick to sensible (that is, 2- to 3-ounce) portions of regular pasta or a slice of organic sourdough bread, and be sure to count them toward your overall daily grain consumption.

10. Legumes: If you want to eat less animal protein, as many people do these days, beans should be right at the top of your shopping list as a great source of protein and fiber. Lentils are my top pick because they cook in less than twenty minutes and they're also a little easier for my body to digest. Experiment with the different varieties; red, brown, green, and black lentils all cook up a little bit differently. I eat them in soups, salads, and grain bowls. See page 90 for information on cooking your own from scratch, which is supersimple—and economical too! Other versatile choices include chickpeas, cannellini beans, or black beans. *Have up to 1 cup per day.*

11. Healthy fats: I'm asked all the time which fats are best to cook with, and most of the time my answer is olive oil—first-pressed evoo for raw uses, like dressing and finishing drizzles, and a less pricey regular olive oil for cooking. I find its earthy, fruity flavor works best with the ingredients I cook with most often, and evoo in particular has the extra bonus of antioxidants. When I'm baking, coconut oil (cold-pressed, virgin oil is less processed) or good European-style butter, preferably made from pasture-raised cow's milk, are my go-tos. In the case of both butter and coconut oil, it pays to buy the best organic, least processed brand you can find. *Have 2 to 4 tablespoons (or half an avocado) per day.*

12. Warm spices: Just about anything you might use to flavor a pumpkin pie qualifies as a warm spice: cinnamon, ginger, and cloves are full of antioxidants as well as delicious flavor. Turmeric, the spice that makes curry powder yellow, is a great inflammation fighter. I find teas and plant-based supplements are sometimes the easiest ways to get these foods in beneficial quantities (see page 66), but I also like to use them to flavor breakfast puddings, stews, and desserts. *Use in unlimited quantities.*

A FEW HELPFUL EXTRAS

When you get ready to cook from this book, your shopping cart isn't going to look very different than it normally would because you will be eating just simple, unprocessed foods—things you can find at any well-stocked supermarket. When it comes to desserts, though, I have found that a handful of ingredients (some of which are relatively new to my pantry) allows me to cook in a way that feels familiar and celebratory without the sugar/dairy/gluten aftermath. Don't worry, it's not a long list; I don't like to run all over town looking for specialty ingredients that cost three times as much as what I used to buy, and I won't ask you to do that either. Stock up once and you will be able to make just about any recipe in this book without making an extra trip to the store.

There are literally dozens of alternative flours and sweeteners available these days, but these are the ones that I find perform consistently well and are moderately priced.

✳ **Rice flour:** Alternatives to wheat flour are common these days, including gluten-free flour blends that include a mixture of corn- or potato starch, xantham gum, and other flours. To keep it simple, all the recipes in this book are made with white rice flour, which is inexpensive and widely available, and/or almond flour. Be sure to get plain rice flour made from long-grain white or brown rice, not glutinous rice flour (also called sweet rice flour), which cooks up dense and chewy.

* **Almond flour:** If your store carries both almond flour and almond meal, choose the former. Almond flour tends to be more finely ground than meal, making it better for baking, and unlike almond meal, most almond flour is made from blanched nuts. That's a benefit because the skins are thought to be harder to digest than the nutmeats themselves.

* **Coconut sugar:** My sweetener of choice these days is coconut sugar. It's less highly refined than cane sugar and, to my palate, a bit less sweet, but it performs well in baking recipes. I use it to sweeten my coffee instead of cane sugar because it's even less processed than the "raw" sugar packets I used to rely on.

* **Coconut yogurt:** When used in sauces, desserts, or breakfast smoothies and parfaits, I prefer the rich texture and clean flavor of coconut yogurt to dairy-free products made from soy or nuts. COYO and Anita's are two brands I have used successfully.

* **Brown rice:** Affordable, widely available, and pleasantly neutral as a bed for just about anything, brown rice is my default grain for breakfast bowls, stir-fries, and more. I like the short-grain

variety because it's stickier and naturally sweeter than its long-grain, but nutty, counterpart brown basmati rice.

* **Chia:** Tiny black chia seeds, either whole or ground into meal, are a terrific source of fiber and omega-3 fatty acids, as well as other essential nutrients, such as protein and calcium. When combined with liquid, they swell and become almost gelatinous, making them a good way to add body to smoothies and thicken puddings and even fruit preserves. Always soak chia seeds before eating to avoid stomach upset.

* **Quinoa:** If you haven't hopped on the quinoa train yet, it's about time! Because it's a seed and not a true grain, quinoa has more protein than grains like rice, oats, and barley, and a nuttier flavor. I like it because it is light and the grains stay separate and fluffy, making it great on its own or as a mixer with other grains and salad greens.

Note: You'll notice there are no nondairy cheeses on this list, because these are often highly processed foods, which I try to avoid. Now that I've reset my gut and have strengthened my immune system, I can eat modest amounts of the real thing without suffering the kind of digestive meltdowns I used to, and I always find that more satisfying than eating "faux" foods in any quantity!

THE REAL SUPERFOODS

"Superfood" is overused these days, and the truth is, no single food has the magical power to keep us healthy—I wish! Some are richer in particular nutrients we can all benefit from, such as omega-3 fatty acids or antioxidants, but the reality is that the quantity you'd need to eat to reap a significant benefit might not be all that appetizing. If you are a fan of blueberries, flaxseeds, or acai berries, by all means add them to your smoothie, but those alone won't promote the kind of healing I'm talking about.

For me, superfoods are ingredients that punch way above their weight when it comes to making things taste, smell, or look amazing, and they do it in a way that won't disturb the balance you're trying to restore in your gut. You probably won't be surprised that a lot of these come straight out of the Italian pantry—there is a reason the Mediterranean diet is acknowledged by doctors around the world as the healthiest.

Feel free to use any of the foods on this list to amp up the flavor of simple, clean ingredients without putting a strain on your recovering gut.

* **Capers:** These salty little nuggets and their larger cousins, caperberries, burst in your mouth and add briny brightness to dressings, tuna salad, pan sauces, and pastas. Fry them in a bit of oil to create crunchy tidbits to top seafood dishes or salads.

* **Olives:** Like capers, olives contribute a tangy salinity to lots of dishes and a meaty mouthfeel that is super satisfying. I prefer green olives to black ones, especially green Castelvetrano olives and Cerignolas, which have an apple-like bite and a clean, briny flavor.

* **Baby arugula:** I probably eat arugula at least once a day! It makes a great counterpoint to richer foods, adds color and freshness in sauces, or works as a bed for anything with a sauce.

* **Fennel:** You can eat unlimited amounts of this crispy bulb vegetable—and I do! It's good cooked or raw, in soups, salads, and stews, or braised all on its own as a side. Substitute it in almost any recipe that calls for chopped celery to add another layer of subtle flavor.

* **Fresh herbs:** Tender herbs like basil, tarragon, mint, and parsley have loads of flavor and in most cases are even more nutritious than salad greens like lettuce. Toss them by the generous handful into vegetable and grain salads or your favorite smoothie, or triple the amount called for in a soup or pasta sauce for a boost of green energy.

✳ **Apple cider vinegar:** A lot of the dressings in this book call for cider vinegar. It's a little sweeter than red wine vinegar and doesn't have the added sugar of commercial balsamic vinegars. Look for an unfiltered, unpasteurized one, which contains gut-friendly bacteria. It gives sauces a bit of acidity when you don't want to add wine or alcohol.

✳ **Lemons:** My love of lemon is well documented, but don't forget about the zest when you are cooking with lemon juice. The little shreds add texture and amplify the lemony flavor of dressings, sauces, and desserts with every bite. The same goes for the zests of limes and oranges.

✳ **Pecorino cheese:** Because it is made from sheep's milk rather than cow's milk, many people find pecorino easier to digest than Parmigiano-Reggiano, and the stronger, sharper flavor means a little goes a long way. (It's also a little easier on the wallet than a good imported Parmigiano-Reggiano.)

✳ **Anchovies:** These tiny fish may be divisive, but in my experience, even folks who claim to hate anchovies love the recipes they star in—after all, who doesn't like a Caesar salad? They are especially effective at waking up the flavors of vegetables like cauliflower and adding an earthy, salty tang when mashed into sauces.

✳ **Tomato paste and sun-dried tomatoes:** Nothing gives sauces, soups, and stews depth of flavor like tomatoes, but you don't need to add a 28-ounce can to the pot to get the benefit. Sautéing a tablespoon or two of tomato paste until it darkens and develops some caramelization is an easy way to pump up flavor in many dishes without making them taste overtly "tomato-y"; two sun-dried tomatoes, finely sliced, do the same for a grain dish or a pan sauce.

✳ **Mushrooms:** Whether in a starring role or as a background player, fresh or dried mushrooms provide body, meaty texture, and earthy flavor. I like dried porcini because they are shelf-stable, and when soaked, they produce a flavorful broth to soups or risottos, as well as yielding tasty mushrooms.

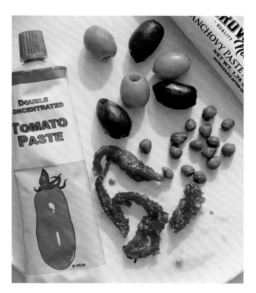

THE BOTTOM LINE

A great meal starts with good ingredients, so try to approach shopping for your food as the first step of every recipe you make, not just a chore to tick off your to-do list. Think about the upcoming week and which situations you'll be in so you can get ahead of the curve, not find yourself stuck with poor choices (see the meal planners in the next chapters for some ideas). If you like to improvise, let what's in season or on sale dictate your menus; I think you'll find many of the recipes in this book flexible enough to adapt to whatever you bring home.

When you are cooking as clean and smart as you will be with these recipes, the quality of your ingredients really matters.

After all, when you're not using a lot of flavor-boosting crutches, like prepared sauces, too-generous amounts of cheese or other dairy, or anything else that fills that metaphorical bucket of doom in your gut, your ingredients can't hide! So take the time to buy the best you can, and treat yourself to a trip to a farmer's market or specialty store now and then.

And take a minute to look at your cart as you're checking out, and reflect on how colorful and fresh and healthy everything looks without all those packaged items you've bought in the past. It's living proof that you've taken a huge step toward a happier gut and a healthier life.

CHAPTER 4

Meal Planning and Menus

You've been cooking and eating a certain way for a long time, and it may take a while before making better choices becomes second nature. In this chapter I'll explain how I think about putting together a week's worth of menus and the basic guidelines to observe when feeding yourself and family. And if you'd rather leave the meal planning to me, I've got you covered with a template for three full weeks of healthy meals that you can adapt to your needs and preferences.

If you hate to be tied to a weekly schedule and prefer to pick and choose your way through this book, that is absolutely fine. I don't always know what I'm going to feel like eating five days down the road either! I do think it's helpful, though, to plan ahead so that you have everything on hand to eat cleanly without falling back on old habits. And using leftovers smartly and ganging your prep work does make the task of cooking more than you may be accustomed to feel a little less daunting.

RESETTING YOUR DIGESTION

By this point you may be champing at the bit to get cooking, and maybe you've already jumped ahead to the recipes and earmarked a few you want to try. If so, by all means, get thee to the kitchen! Encouraging you to integrate a few—or a lot—of these recipes into your repertoire is my main goal. But to feel the full benefits of this approach to cooking, recipes like these should be the rule rather than the exception, especially if they represent a significant change to the way you are used to eating.

Nowadays I eat this way *most* of the time, especially during the week, when I do a lot of my own cooking. On the weekends, though, I give myself a little more latitude. That way I can socialize, eat at other people's homes, or go to restaurants without having to make special requests. In the long run I have found that eating really well 70 to 80 percent of the time keeps my energy level high, my immunity strong, and my digestive system on a sufficiently even keel that it can cope with the occasional slice of three-cheese pizza or an ice cream sundae without too much trouble. I may not feel 100 percent when Monday rolls around, but it doesn't take me long to bounce back, and I never suffer the kind of full-body exhaustion and brain fog that used to follow me. Giving myself that kind of flexibility on weekends also makes my cleaner Monday-through-Friday routine feel a lot more doable.

If you really want to see how eating better affects your digestion and overall well-being, try eating according to the following principles (or using the meal plans) for twenty-one days. Psychologists say it takes twenty-one days to form a new habit—or, in this case, to change your dietary habits. In those three weeks you will also be able to reset your system gently by minimizing foods that cause stress and inflammation in favor of cleaner, more gut-friendly options. After that period you can segue into the kind of 80/20 approach that works for me and start to reintroduce some of the foods

you've been steering clear of—if you want to. You will probably get some feedback from your gut on what makes it happy and what doesn't; use that information to help you plan out your meals going forward.

GIADA'S CHEAT SHEET

* Aim to have a leafy green (cooked or raw) as a part of at least two meals every day.
* Go for four or five ½-cup servings of vegetables daily.
* Limit carb-based meals like pasta, grain bowls, potatoes, or starchy breakfasts like pancakes or oatmeal to one per day.
* Limit animal proteins (excluding eggs) to one meal per day *at most*.
* Have one or two vegetarian days each week.
* Use alternative protein sources such as eggs, seeds and nuts, legumes, or quinoa for one meal per day.
* Limit desserts or alcohol to two servings total per week.
* Confine dairy consumption to ½ cup over the course of a day, including Parmigiano-Reggiano and butter, and don't have it every day.

Here are a few guidelines that I like to think about as I plan my meals for the day.

Eat these foods infrequently—no more than twice per week.

* Red meat (including beef, lamb, or pork)

* Processed foods

* Dairy

* Wheat (as in flour or in other forms, including whole grains or bulgur)

As a rule, I try to minimize the role prepared or processed foods play in my diet—down to seemingly benign products like packaged nut milks and chicken broth. Even pasta falls into this category, as do bottled sauces and convenience foods like bagels and frozen waffles (both of which also contain wheat, another ingredient I avoid when possible). If this feels unrealistic for you (and if so, no judgment), be sure you choose the options with the shortest ingredient lists and the fewest additives.

Meat is another food I have scaled way, way back on, in both frequency and portion size. I aim for servings of protein—including lean protein like fish and chicken—that are about the size of my palm. For me, that means no more than 4 to 6 ounces and frequently even less if it's a rich meat like pork or beef.

Last, dairy shows up less and less often on my menus, and when it does, I use it primarily as a flavor enhancer (think Parmigiano-Reggiano, feta, or occasionally goat cheese) rather than the star ingredient.

Eat from this category in moderation— aim for a single serving from any three of these categories per day.

* Sustainable fish like salmon, shrimp, and sardines

* Poultry

* Eggs

* Low-glycemic fruits, particularly berries, as well as apples, stone fruits, and cherries

* Legumes like lentils, cannellini beans, and chickpeas

* Starchy vegetables like carrots, squash, peas, and green beans

* Sweet potatoes

* Root vegetables like turnips, potatoes, and beets

* Nuts, seeds, and peanuts, whole or ground

* Whole, unprocessed grains like brown rice, millet, and quinoa

* Foods high in fat (even "good" fats such as avocado and evoo), like coconut and cheese

Even though these all make the Delectable Dozen list (page 32), to feel my best, I try to limit the number of meals these foods appear in as well as the quantities I eat over the course of a day. Take grains, for example. If I have pancakes or French toast for breakfast, I don't have a rice bowl for lunch or pasta for dinner; I'll save those for a day when I had a smoothie or eggs for breakfast and a big salad at lunch. And I don't go overboard on animal protein either. I make sure that one of my main meals, either lunch or dinner, is meatless every day, and often I have no meat—including fish and poultry—at all.

As a rule of thumb, think about choosing a maximum of three items from these categories each day (I limit the serving size to a cup or less), perhaps having berries in your smoothie and a bit of grain or beans with your lunch. Follow my meal plans for a few days, and you'll get the hang of it.

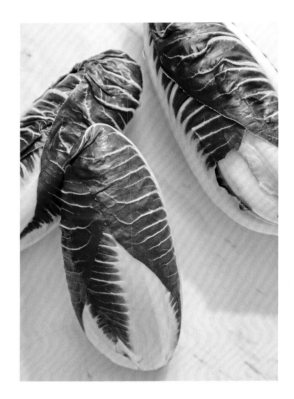

Eat to your heart's (and gut's) content— no restriction on quantity.

* Dark leafy greens like kale, chard, collards

* Cruciferous veggies like cauliflower, broccoli, broccoli rabe, Brussels sprouts, cabbage

* Salad veggies (radishes, cucumbers, celery) and salad greens

* Tender veggies like asparagus, zucchini, fennel

Greens, tender veggies, and more greens are the starting point for the majority of my meals. They don't need to be the main event; think of them as extenders or additions to the dishes you already eat. Throw some spinach into a chicken dish, stir some arugula into a risotto, roast some broccoli along with your sheet pan dinner. If you have roasted veggies or sautéed greens in the fridge, add them to a pasta sauce, tuck them into a sandwich, or use them to build a grain bowl with a little bit of protein (beans, leftover chicken) and some sliced avocado. Get it?

TRICKS OF THE TRADE

Over the years I've picked up some strategies for incorporating these new food realities into my lifestyle more easily and seamlessly. I find they are simple ways to make sure I'm prioritizing the foods I want to eat more of—and painless ways to minimize those I don't. And you don't need to be a chef to pull off any of these, promise.

✳ **Batch it up:** I started cooking this way when I first had my daughter, Jade, because as a sleep-deprived new parent I rarely had the wherewithal to cook a whole meal from scratch. Cooking batches of simple ingredients while she was napping and storing them in the fridge allowed me to pull together easy meals almost instantly; now it's become as much a part of my weekly routine as shopping. I'm such an advocate of batch cooking I've devoted a whole chapter to these plug-and-play components; see pages 76–102 for some of my favorite foods to batch up.

✳ **Swap it out:** Whenever I am about to reach for something on the Proceed with Caution list, I ask myself if there is a healthier way to achieve a similar result. Here are a few favorites:

　» Serve fish or meat on a bed of undressed baby arugula or other greens instead of mashed potatoes, rice, or polenta. They will soak up the juices and give you an extra helping of greens to boot.

　» For a special dinner, serve lamb or a beautiful salmon fillet instead of the more expected beef entrée. You can serve them with just about any sauce you'd put on a steak (try the Scallion Salsa Verde on page 209) for a steakhouse-style meal, with far less saturated fat and nasty additives.

　» Substitute almond flour or rice flour for bread crumbs or panko in breaded dishes and meat loaf.

　» Pan-braise vegetables or mushrooms in a bit of broth instead of sautéing or stir-frying in oil; finish with a bit of butter or a drizzle of evoo for flavor just before serving.

　» Choose dry, aged cheeses over soft cheeses; many people feel the aging process makes these cheeses more digestible. Goat's and sheep's milk dairy products can also be easier to process for people with dairy sensitivities.

　» Try coconut milk or coconut yogurt as a substitute for cream, yogurt, or sour cream.

✳ **Turn it upside down:** If there's a meal you or your family can't live without, see if you can play with the ratio of veggies

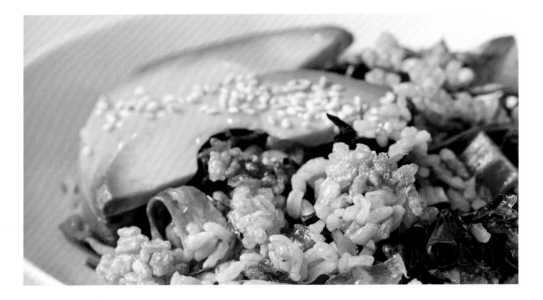

to protein or carbs to make it better for your digestion. For example, double up on the clams (or stretch them with bits of shrimp or calamari) and use just half a box of pasta when you make linguine and clam sauce; serve chicken Parm over lightly dressed greens instead of on a hero roll (and bread the chicken using almond flour or rice flour); sub in diced zucchini, fennel, and carrots for half the meat in your Bolognese sauce.

* **Serve it up in a bowl:** There's something supercozy and intimate about food served in a bowl. The food effortlessly looks more artful and composed than when it's all spread across a plate, both casual and elegant at the same time. Without so much real estate to fill up, it's easier to control portions too. I like to use a shallow pasta-style bowl for just about everything, from noodles to soups to salads to steak.

* **Think like a food stylist:** When you use a special ingredient, make a little go a long way by showing it off. Toss your salad first before shaving a few big shards of Parm or pecorino on top for maximum impact. Grate a little bit of bittersweet chocolate onto a fruit parfait to make it seem decadent. Sprinkle nuts on top of your baked goods rather than stirring them into the batter so they get more toasty and crunchy. You don't need to use more—in fact you can probably use less—but you'll get more bang for your buck.

A FINAL NOTE:
EATING OUT AND
EATING AWAY FROM HOME

It's possible to maintain the great gut situation you've finally achieved if you think a little outside the box. Start by choosing a restaurant that you know will have some reasonable options for you; Italian, Greek, and Middle Eastern restaurants all tend to have lots of vegetable dishes and prepare their proteins simply, without a lot of heavy sauces.

*   Make your own entrée by ordering two or three vegetable sides.

*   Ask if you can substitute a salad (evoo and lemon on the side) for fried or starchy side dishes.

*   If you're having two courses, order an app for both, or split an entrée with a friend.

*   Ask for a box and take home half your entrée for lunch the next day; most restaurant portions are more than enough for two meals, especially if you serve your leftovers over a salad.

*   Don't overdo it on the booze. Order a spritzer or something relatively clean and made without sugary mixers, and ask for extra ice to extend it (see right).

*   Order a couple of desserts for the table and have just a bite or two.

Don't be afraid to ask for what you want; these days most restaurants are eager to accommodate the needs of their customers, especially if you ask politely. And if there truly aren't any great options on the menu, try not to fret or let it spoil the evening. The real point is to enjoy spending time with your friends, not to be perfect. It's just one meal out of one day, and the choices you've been making the rest of the time will stand you in good stead when you find yourself in a situation where you just *have* to eat a plate of fried chicken. Tomorrow is always another day.

WHAT ABOUT ALCOHOL

When I'm in a social situation or somewhere everyone else is drinking, I usually have a glass of either Prosecco or white wine with a few ice cubes. I know wine snobs will roll their eyes, but the ice dilutes the alcohol and also makes the drink last longer. My mom has used this trick for years, and now I do too. It lets me be part of the party without imbibing more than I want to.

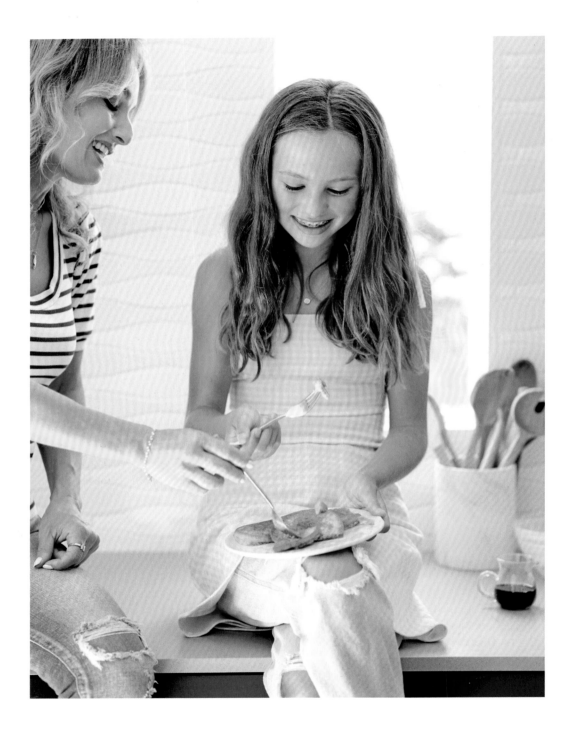

CHAPTER 5

The Meal Plans

Using preplanned menus makes it easier for some people to stay on the straight and narrow while they are getting comfortable with a new cooking strategy. If that's you, you'll find this three-week plan—a mixture of recipes from throughout the book supplemented with easy improvised meals from the prefab elements in the batch cooking chapter—will help you get in a good groove. Even if you'd rather freestyle your own meal plans, I suggest you check out these menus to get a better idea of how to prioritize gut-supporting foods over those that send you down the road to poor health.

To get the greatest benefit from these recipes, I urge you to commit to using them—and only them—for three full weeks. During these twenty-one days, you will be creating maximum space for healing, and devoting less time to recovery, so desserts are limited to gluten-free, homemade treats, and foods from the Proceed with Caution list are very limited. If you have alcohol, limit it to one or two servings per week.

The following plan is an example of what three full weeks of superclean eating looks like. It assumes you will be cooking for two or fewer, as in many cases leftovers from one meal are rolled over into a new

meal another day. Several of the recipes within each weekly plan make strategic use of the items you will have batch-cooked in preparation for the upcoming week, both in the recipes and for the "improv" meals you will be pulling together. In addition to the pre-prepped grain, veggies, and protein you need for each of the three weeks in this plan, I also suggest you get ready for this 3-week stretch by stirring up a double batch of your favorite vinaigrette, some Kale Pesto (page 89), plenty of broth and cooked proteins (pages 95 and 96), and a few hard-boiled eggs, and replenish them as needed. If you haven't already, bake some Maple and Olive Oil Quinoa Granola (page 114) for snacking and adding crunch to breakfasts.

After twenty-one days, putting together a week's worth of meals and coming up with new ways to reuse and refresh your batched items and leftovers will become second nature. It may even make you a more creative (and economical) cook. And once you know how good eating this way makes you feel, you may never want to go back to your old "favorites" again. Use the lists on pages 54 to 55 to stock your shelves and fridge.

IMPROV MEALS

You'll notice that many of the lunches in these meal plans, as well as an occasional dinner, are designated as IMPROV meals (and labeled as such). That means you won't find a specific recipe for them in this book. Instead, I'm suggesting that you use the prepped ingredients from your batch cooking (page 78) together with some pantry items or leftovers from previous meals to assemble a recipe-free soup, salad, or grain bowl that requires minimal or no cooking. Reheat cooked grains in the microwave and

arrange warmed or room temperature ingredients on top—drizzled with some pesto, Scallion Salsa Verde (page 209) or vinaigrette if you like—for an easy IMPROV grain bowl. (Adding a few slices of avocado never hurts!) For an IMPROV soup, simmer raw or cooked greens and veggies in hot broth just until warmed through or wilted. Add a teeny drizzle of your best extra-virgin olive oil and a dollop of pesto or a sprinkle of grated Parmigiano-Reggiano and you have a fast and fresh-tasting soup in five minutes or less. IMPROV salads are even easier; just toss almost anything in the fridge with a splash of vinaigrette and

Week 1

PREP DAY: Vegetable or chicken broth (page 95 or 96) | Maple and Olive Oil Quinoa Granola (page 114) | Sautéed greens (page 86) | White beans (page 90) | Kale Pesto (page 89)

	DAY 1	DAY 2	DAY 3
BREAKFAST	Maple and Olive Oil Quinoa Granola (page 114) with Almond Milk (page 104)	Smoothie (pages 105–108)	Coconut Yogurt Parfait (page 112) or leftover smoothie (from day 2)
LUNCH	IMPROV soup: Hot broth ladled over sautéed greens, white beans, Kale Pesto	IMPROV salad: Leftover Parmesan shrimp and a few sweet potato wedges (both from day 1) on baby arugula and kale	White Bean and Escarole Soup (page 141), Mista Salad with Roasted Garlic Dressing (page 220)
DINNER	Sheet Pan Parmesan Shrimp and Veggies (page 202), Gigi's Sweet Potato Wedges (page 227)	Green Fried Rice (page 142), simple salad	IMPROV grain bowl: Leftover Green Fried Rice (from day 2) topped with sautéed greens, Kale Pesto, and a fried egg

serve over greens, maybe bolstered with a quartered hard-boiled egg. You'll find a half dozen great dressings on pages 150–164 (I'm partial to the Raspberry Dressing on page 159) or keep it super easy with a squeeze of lemon juice, a drizzle of your very best evoo, and a sprinkle of flake salt. Unleash your inner *Chopped* champion and use what you have to make a fast and fresh meal that will rival anything you would get from that salad chain or fast-casual spot you've come to rely on (and at a fraction of the cost).

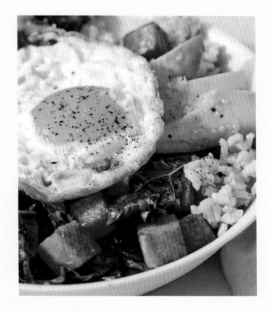

Remember: These menus assume you are cooking for two and saving two portions for future meals.

DAY 4	DAY 5	DAY 6	DAY 7
Warm Quinoa "Oatmeal" (page 120)	Olive Oil–Scrambled Eggs (page 115)	Buckwheat Cardamom Pancakes (page 124) or Quinoa Pancakes (page 123)	Mushroom Toast (page 119)
IMPROV salad: Chopped veggies, avocado, and greens with a sprinkle of chopped nuts	Leftover White Bean and Escarole Soup (from day 3), half portion of last night's salmon (day 4) over greens with Kale Pesto	IMPROV soup: Shredded Amalfi Lemon Chicken (from day 5) and chopped greens in broth with a sprinkle of pecorino	IMPROV salad: Leftover roasted broccoli (from day 6), white beans, roasted potatoes (from day 6), and raw greens and veggies
Broiled Salmon with Crushed Broccoli (page 217), Green Bean "Fries" (page 228)	Amalfi Lemon Chicken (page 189), Escarole and Olive Salad with Raspberry Dressing (page 159)	Pan-Roasted Pork Chops with Cherry and Red Wine Sauce (page 210), Crispy Roasted Broccoli (page 224), Herbes de Provence Roasted Potatoes (page 223)	Artichoke and Brussels Sprout Brown Rice Risotto (page 184), Aqua Pazza (page 201), mixed salad

Week 2

PREP DAY: Breakfast Chia Seed Pudding (page 111) | Big Batch Roasted Veggies (page 83) | A Lotta Lentils (page 91) | Big Batch Brown Rice (page 94)

	DAY 8	DAY 9	DAY 10
BREAKFAST	Breakfast Chia Seed Pudding	Smoothie (pages 105–108)	Breakfast Chia Seed Pudding
LUNCH	Roasted Cauliflower and Baby Kale Salad (page 153) on a bed of lentils	Leftover fusilli (from day 8), mixed salad	Creamy Cauliflower Soup with Pepitas (page 134), green salad
DINNER	Fusilli with Pesto and Green Beans (page 170)	Easy Chicken Piccata (page 194), roasted veggies, Curry-Roasted Butternut Squash (page 238)	Spiced Sweet Potato Rice Bowl with Fried Egg (page 145)

Week 3

PREP DAY: Lemon and Oregano Pounded Chicken (page 99) | Basic Boccoli Rabe (page 85) | Vegetable or chicken broth (page 95 or 96) | Big Batch Quinoa (page 92) | Hard-Boiled Eggs Two Ways (page 132)

	DAY 15	DAY 16	DAY 17
BREAKFAST	Reheated pancakes (from day 14)	Smoothie (pages 105–108) or Green Refresher (page 128)	Olive Oil–Scrambled Eggs with Arugula and Fennel Salad (page 115)
LUNCH	Red, White, and Blue Salad (page 164)	Leftover Red, White, and Blue Salad (from day 15), quartered hard-boiled egg	IMPROV salad: Sliced pounded chicken over baby kale with crumbled feta
DINNER	IMPROV grain bowl: Warm quinoa and broccoli rabe with a fried egg	Quinoa and Sweet Potato Stew-ish (page 138)	Salad, Spaghetti with Rosemary and Lemon (page 169)

Remember: These menus assume you are cooking for two
and saving two portions for future meals.

DAY 11	DAY 12	DAY 13	DAY 14
Asparagus Scramble (page 116)	Smoothie (pages 105–108)	Warm Quinoa "Oatmeal" (page 120)	Quinoa or Buckwheat Cardamom Pancakes (page 123–124; freeze leftovers)
IMPROV salad: Leftover Easy Chicken Piccata (from day 9) over arugula	Leftover sweet potato rice bowl (from day 10) with roasted veggies	IMPROV grain bowl: Leftover salmon (from day 12) and raw veggies on brown rice drizzled with Kale Pesto (page 89)	Leftover stuffed squash (from day 13), mixed salad
Steamed Cod with Coconut Broth (page 146) over brown rice	Broiled Salmon and Fennel Salad (page 150) on a bed of lentils	Lentil-Stuffed Squash (page 205)	Grilled Strip Steak with Scallion Salsa Verde (page 209), Fennel-Roasted Yukon Golds (page 240)

Remember: These menus assume you are cooking for two
and saving two portions for future meals.

DAY 18	DAY 19	DAY 20	DAY 21
Smoothie (pages 105–108) or Green Refresher (page 128)	Coconut Yogurt Parfait (page 112)	Reheated pancakes (from day 14)	Asparagus Scramble (page 116) with smoked salmon
IMPROV soup: Quinoa with broth, chopped broccoli rabe, and chopped pounded chicken	Leftover stew-ish (from day 16), simple salad	IMPROV soup: Leftover Cauliflower–Sweet Potato Mash (from day 19) thinned and pureed with broth until smooth, then topped with chopped herbs or nuts	IMPROV salad: Hard-Boiled Eggs Two Ways (page 132) over baby greens, sliced celery, and sliced fennel
Roasted Trout with Hazelnut Gremolata (page 198), Grilled Wedge Salad (page 156)	Lamb Chops with Mint and Pistachio Salsa Verde (page 215), Cauliflower–Sweet Potato Mash (page 241)	Sole with Lemon-Caper Sauce (page 195), Simple Salad of Bitter Greens (page 218)	Chicken Milanese (page 190), quinoa, Creamy Dill Coleslaw (page 219)

STAPLES

- [ ] Olive oil
- [ ] Coconut oil
- [ ] Dark sesame oil
- [ ] Apple cider vinegar
- [ ] Champagne vinegar
- [ ] Dijon mustard
- [ ] Whole-grain mustard

- [ ] French or green lentils
- [ ] Dried cannellini beans
- [ ] Short-grain brown rice
- [ ] Long-grain brown rice
- [ ] White quinoa
- [ ] Local honey
- [ ] Pure maple syrup

- [ ] Tamari
- [ ] Dark sesame oil
- [ ] Capers in brine
- [ ] Calabrian chile paste
- [ ] Kosher salt
- [ ] Flake salt
- [ ] Bay leaves

- [ ] Red pepper flakes
- [ ] Dried oregano
- [ ] Groud cinnamon
- [ ] Pure vanilla extract
- [ ] Black peppercorns

WEEK 1 *(includes pre-prep)*

PRODUCE

- [ ] Smoothie ingredients for the week
- [ ] Pancake ingredients for the week
- [ ] 1 lime
- [ ] 7 lemons
- [ ] 3 heads garlic
- [ ] 1 knob ginger
- [ ] 4 shallots
- [ ] 3 onions
- [ ] 2 red onions
- [ ] 1 pint cherry tomatoes
- [ ] 1 bag carrots
- [ ] 1 head celery
- [ ] 2 avocados
- [ ] 1 pound assorted mushrooms
- [ ] 4 heads broccoli
- [ ] 1 medium cauliflower
- [ ] 2 bunches asparagus
- [ ] ½ pound green beans
- [ ] 1 Yukon Gold potato
- [ ] 24 ounces golden Peewee potatoes
- [ ] 3 small sweet potatoes
- [ ] 1 bunch thyme
- [ ] 1 bunch rosemary
- [ ] 1 bunch basil
- [ ] 1 bunch scallions

- [ ] 1 bunch chives
- [ ] 1 bunch Italian parsley
- [ ] 3 fennel bulbs
- [ ] 10 ounces Brussels sprouts
- [ ] 2 bunches Tuscan kale
- [ ] 1 bunch Swiss chard
- [ ] 2 heads Treviso or radicchio
- [ ] 1 head Bibb lettuce
- [ ] 3 small heads escarole
- [ ] 2 (5-ounce) containers baby kale
- [ ] 1 (5-ounce) container baby spinach
- [ ] 1 (5-ounce) container baby arugula
- [ ] 1 (5-ounce) container mesclun mix
- [ ] 3 half-pints raspberries
- [ ] 1 pint blueberries

DRY GOODS

- [ ] 1 (32-ounce) carton unsweetened almond milk
- [ ] 1 (14-ounce) can cherry tomatoes
- [ ] 1 jar herbes de Provence
- [ ] 1 jar Old Bay seasoning
- [ ] 9 ounces walnut halves

- [ ] 10 ounces raw almonds
- [ ] 6 ounces pitted dates
- [ ] 2 ounces tart dried cherries
- [ ] 1 cup mixed olives
- [ ] 1 (8-ounce) container gluten-free bread crumbs
- [ ] 1 loaf rustic bread or other gluten-free panko bread

DAIRY

- [ ] ½ pound unsalted European-style butter
- [ ] ¼-pound wedge Parmigiano-Reggiano
- [ ] ¼-pound wedge Pecorino Romano
- [ ] 2 (5.3-ounce) containers coconut yogurt or 2% Greek yogurt
- [ ] 1 dozen eggs
- [ ] 2-ounce piece Gorgonzola dolce (optional)

PROTEIN

- [ ] 2 whole chickens (about 3½ pounds each)
- [ ] 1 pound large shrimp, peeled and deveined

- [ ] 4 cod fillets (about 5 ounces each)
- [ ] 1 (1½-inch thick) NY strip steak (1¾ pounds total)
- [ ] 1 wild king salmon piece (about 1 pound)
- [ ] 4 center-cut salmon fillets (about 5 ounces each)
- [ ] 4 skinless striped bass fillets (about 6 ounces each)
- [ ] 2 thick bone-in pork loin chops (10 to 12 ounces each)

FROZEN

- [ ] 1 (8-ounce) bag cherries
- [ ] 6 ounces frozen artichoke hearts

ALCOHOL

- [ ] 1 bottle dry marsala
- [ ] 1 bottle dry red wine, such as Pinot Noir
- [ ] 1 bottle dry white wine, such as Pinot Grigio

WEEK 2 (includes pre-prep)

PRODUCE

- [ ] Smoothie ingredients for the week
- [ ] Pancake ingredients for the week
- [ ] 2 pints blueberries
- [ ] 1 bunch red grapes
- [ ] 1 mango
- [ ] 1 lemon
- [ ] 2 limes
- [ ] 1 red onion
- [ ] 5 shallots
- [ ] 1 avocado
- [ ] 2 heads garlic
- [ ] 1 knob ginger
- [ ] 1 pint cherry tomatoes
- [ ] 1 serrano pepper
- [ ] 1 head celery
- [ ] 1 bunch radishes
- [ ] ½ pound green beans
- [ ] 1 head broccoli
- [ ] 3 heads cauliflower
- [ ] 3 small sweet potatoes
- [ ] 2 large Yukon Gold potatoes (about 1 pound total)

- [ ] 3 delicata squash
- [ ] 1 butternut squash
- [ ] 2 fennel bulbs
- [ ] 1 bunch thyme
- [ ] 1 bunch Italian parsley
- [ ] 3 bunches basil
- [ ] 1 bunch cilantro
- [ ] 1 bunch oregano
- [ ] 2 bunches scallions
- [ ] 1 bunch asparagus
- [ ] 2 bunches Tuscan kale
- [ ] 1 (5-ounce) container baby kale
- [ ] 2 (5-ounce) containers baby arugula
- [ ] 1 (5-ounce) container mesclun mix
- [ ] 1 (5-ounce) container baby spinach

DRY GOODS

- [ ] 1 jar za'atar
- [ ] 1 jar ground cardamom
- [ ] 1 jar curry powder
- [ ] 1 jar ground turmeric
- [ ] 1 jar smoked paprika

- [ ] 1 jar pumpkin pie spice
- [ ] 1 tube anchovy paste
- [ ] 1 (32-ounce) carton unsweetened almond milk
- [ ] ½ cup (about 4 ounces) chia seeds
- [ ] Quinoa flakes
- [ ] 4 ounces walnut halves
- [ ] 3 ounces Marcona almonds
- [ ] 2 ounces pumpkin seeds
- [ ] 2 ounces pine nuts
- [ ] 1 (13.5-ounce) can light coconut milk
- [ ] 1 ounce unsweetened coconut chips
- [ ] ½ pound gluten-free fusilli
- [ ] 1 (32-ounce) carton reduced-sodium chicken broth
- [ ] 1 (32-ounce) carton reduced-sodium vegetable broth

DAIRY

- [ ] 6 ounces feta cheese
- [ ] ¼-pound wedge Parmigiano-Reggiano
- [ ] 1 (15-ounce) container ricotta cheese
- [ ] ½ pound unsalted European-style butter
- [ ] 1 dozen eggs

PROTEIN

- [ ] 4 boneless, skinless chicken breasts (6 ounces each)
- [ ] 4 cod fillets (about 5 ounces each)
- [ ] 1 (1½-inch-thick) NY strip steak (1¾ pounds total)
- [ ] 1 wild king salmon fillet (about 1 pound)

FROZEN

- [ ] 1 (10-ounce) bag frozen peas

WEEK 3 (includes pre-prep)

PRODUCE

- [ ] Smoothie ingredients for the week
- [ ] Pancake ingredients for the week
- [ ] 8 lemons
- [ ] 1 orange
- [ ] 1 bunch red grapes
- [ ] 1 pint blueberries
- [ ] 2 onions
- [ ] 2 heads garlic
- [ ] 1 bag carrots
- [ ] 1 head celery (if needed)
- [ ] 1 avocado
- [ ] 2 fennel bulbs
- [ ] 1 bunch asparagus
- [ ] 1 (8-ounce) package cremini mushrooms
- [ ] 1 delicata squash
- [ ] 1 head cauliflower
- [ ] 1 large Korean sweet potato (about 1 pound)

- [ ] 1 small sweet potato
- [ ] 1 English cucumber
- [ ] 1 bunch thyme
- [ ] 1 bunch chives
- [ ] 1 bunch rosemary
- [ ] 1 bunch oregano
- [ ] 1 bunch basil
- [ ] 2 bunches Italian parsley
- [ ] 1 bunch dill
- [ ] 1 bunch mint
- [ ] 1 bunch broccoli rabe
- [ ] 1 head savoy cabbage
- [ ] 4 heads radicchio
- [ ] 2 small endives
- [ ] 1 head Treviso
- [ ] 2 hearts of romaine or small romaine lettuces
- [ ] 1 bunch collards or kale
- [ ] 1 curly endive or frisée
- [ ] 2 (5-ounce) containers baby arugula

- [ ] 1 (5-ounce) container baby kale

DRY GOODS

- [ ] 1 jar ground cumin
- [ ] 1 jar onion powder
- [ ] 1 jar garlic powder
- [ ] 1 jar cayenne pepper
- [ ] 2 ounces hazelnuts
- [ ] 1 pound spaghetti (gluten-free or regular)
- [ ] 4 ounces pitted mixed olives
- [ ] 6 ounces roasted, lightly salted pistachios
- [ ] 1 bag rice flour
- [ ] 1 (32-ounce) reduced-sodium chicken broth
- [ ] 4 ounces smoked almonds

DAIRY

- [ ] 2 dozen eggs
- [ ] ½ pound unsalted European-style butter
- [ ] ¼-pound piece Gorgonzola dolce
- [ ] ¼-pound wedge Pecorino Romano
- [ ] 1 (6-ounce) container 2% Greek yogurt
- [ ] 1 (27-ounce) container coconut yogurt

PROTEIN

- [ ] 8 boneless, skinless chicken breasts
- [ ] 1 whole chicken
- [ ] 4 rainbow trout fillets
- [ ] 4 sole fillets
- [ ] 12 frenched rib lamb chops
- [ ] 4 ounces smoked salmon

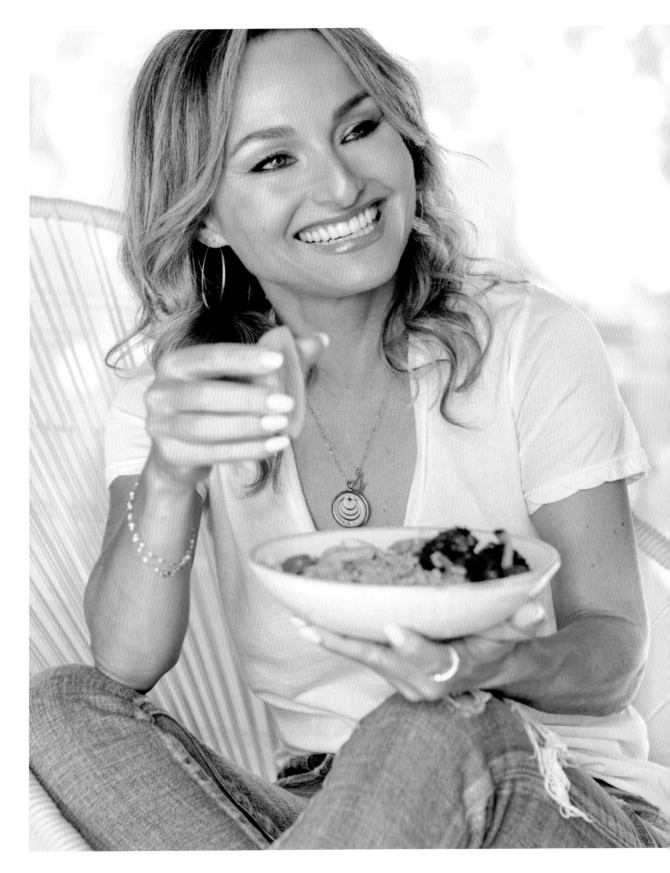

CHAPTER 6

The Reboot: A Three-Day Mini-Cleanse

You know how you can be working on your computer and everything seems to be operating at half speed—or even comes to a complete standstill? Sometimes the only way to get things up and running again is to reboot the whole system.

Well, your digestion is not all that different. When that happens to me, either because I've been too careless about what I'm eating or traveling a lot and eating on an unpredictable schedule, I use a quick reboot plan to get everything back on track. This means giving my gut as much of a break from low-grade inflammation as I possibly can and eating even cleaner and lighter than usual.

When I'm rebooting I eat mostly vegetables and some lean protein, and not too many grains or fruits—about ½ cup of each per day. It keeps me full enough so I have the energy to function and think clearly while giving my digestive system some serious downtime.

I'm not even going to pretend that I eat this way all the time, or that for me it is sustainable over the long haul—I miss my pasta and desserts too much. But it does help me get things moving again if my digestion isn't humming along as it should be. Fortunately, when you eat this clean and simply, you start to see and feel a difference after just a few days. It's also a great way to kick-start your transition to a new, healthier way of eating.

In fact, rebooting makes me feel so good that I do it at least twice a year, usually right after the holidays in January, and then again when I get back from my annual summer vacation, when I tend to indulge in a lot more trips to the ice cream shop, bakery, and pizza parlor than I probably should. If I'm really feeling the effects of having wandered off the straight and narrow, I might extend the reboot for four or five days.

Rebooting is easiest if you do it at a time when you have a fair amount of control over when and what you eat (that means no restaurants or social gatherings, where food choices are limited) and you can plan your meals in advance so you are never caught without a good option. You can choose any three-day stretch that works best for you and your schedule, but I like to reboot Monday through Wednesday. That way I can spend Sunday doing any necessary shopping as well as the prep for a few meals—a few batches of grains or beans, sautéed or roasted veggies, and maybe some grilled chicken or roasted salmon. Come Monday, I'm good to go with easy meals to pack and tote or just throw together right from the fridge. By the time the end of the week rolls around, if I'm meeting up with friends, I'm ready to ease back into my regular eating routine.

HERE'S A LIST OF THE FOODS TO AVOID FOR THE DURATION OF YOUR REBOOT

* All processed food, and most things that come in a package. This means no bars, no protein powders, no pasta (regular or gluten-free). Avoid any canned or jarred goods that contain sugar, stabilizers, or ingredients besides water or salt.

* Red meat, including pork (and pork products like bacon), lamb, and veal.

* Dairy of any kind, including nondairy substitutes other than homemade.

* No more than 1 teaspoon per day of added sugar in any form, including agave, coconut sugar, honey, maple syrup, or any other sneaky stand-ins.

* Baked goods, desserts, and sweets, including ones that are gluten-free.

* High-glycemic fruits, including grapes, pineapple, watermelon, and bananas (some low-glycemic fruits, like berries, are OK in moderation).

* Nightshade vegetables (including tomatoes, potatoes, and peppers).

* Starchy vegetables, such as potatoes and peas.

* More than 2 tablespoons of nuts or raw, unsweetened butter (though healthful, they're hard for the gut to break down), but homemade or additive-free, unflavored nut milk is OK.

* Large quantities of fatty foods like avocado and coconut, which are also harder to digest; no more than ¼ avocado per day.

* Spicy foods, which can cause acid stomach.

* Alcohol.

* Caffeine, except for a single cup a day. I can't live without a cup of coffee or tea in the morning, so I don't expect you to either. But drink it first thing, without dairy or sweetener, and if you don't need it, skip it, because coffee is acidic and therefore can irritate your stomach.

SO WHAT *CAN* YOU EAT?

While you are rebooting, greens and vegetables; eggs, fish, and chicken; low-glycemic fruits; and whole grains like brown rice, quinoa, and millet will be the foundation of your diet. Use the meal plan on page 61, or make your own, choosing from among any of the recipes with a (RB) icon to make your own reboot menus. You can also keep it even more low key by using components from the batch cooking chapter (page 78) to create basic mix-and-match salads, soups, and grain bowls, supplemented by any of the flavor boosters on page 38, except those containing dairy or nuts.

YOU CAN EAT THESE FOODS FOR BREAKFAST, LUNCH, OR DINNER

* Dark leafy greens: kale; Swiss chard; escarole; collards; beet, mustard, or turnip greens; dandelion greens

* Bitter greens and lettuces: arugula, radicchio, Belgian endive, Treviso, frisée, watercress, romaine, Boston lettuce

* Fresh herbs: basil, parsley, dill, cilantro (but not mint, which can cause heartburn)

* Cruciferous vegetables: broccoli, broccoli rabe, cabbage, Brussels sprouts

* Tender vegetables: fennel, asparagus, celery, zucchini

* Alliums: onions, leeks, garlic, shallots

* Herbal teas or infusions (see my Detox Tea on page 74)

HAVE THESE FOODS LESS OFTEN—IDEALLY ONCE PER DAY

* Eggs

* Orange vegetables: carrots, butternut or acorn squash, sweet potatoes

* Fish or lean poultry like chicken breast or ground turkey

* Whole, unrefined grains: brown rice, millet, quinoa

* Legumes like lentils or white beans, preferably freshly cooked, in moderation.

* Good fats, like avocado and olive oil, but only in moderation

If this seems limited, well, it is! Doing a reboot isn't about variety or culinary creativity (though it is still possible to eat deliciously!). This three-day cleanse is really about getting back to basics and eating more simply than we do most of the time in order to allow the gut to start healing. I think of it as going old-school, like spending a few days without your phone or laptop to give your eyes and brain a chance to refocus and recharge. While you are rebooting, you'll probably have less variety than usual, and that's OK. Remember, it's just three days. You can do this!

Rebooting: The Essentials

Whether you use this meal plan or create your own, here are the guidelines for a reboot:

*   Try to eat some cooked or raw greens at every meal.

*   In addition to the greens, have 1 to 2 cups of nonstarchy veggies like broccoli, asparagus, fennel, cauliflower, or Brussels sprouts per day.

*   Limit fruit to one ½-cup serving per day, and choose a low-glycemic variety like berries or stone fruits.

*   Limit grains to ½ cup per *day* (not per meal) and eat only whole grains like brown rice, millet, and quinoa—nothing made from ground grains or flour.

*   Limit beans (fresh or dried) to ½ cup per day.

*   Limit animal protein like fish or chicken to a single meal per day. Eggs may be eaten at another meal in addition to your serving of protein or as a snack.

*   You may *add* a green salad—lettuce, chicories, shaved Brussels sprouts, kale, spinach, and so on, dressed with lemon and a drizzle of evoo (and by a drizzle I mean a teaspoon or two)—to any meal, or use it as a bed for any protein.

*   You can *substitute* any mix-and-match mashup from the batch cooking chapter (page 78) for any breakfast, lunch, or dinner as long as your total grain consumption doesn't exceed ½ cup per day.

*   You can *eliminate* any snack if you're not feeling the need for it, but I find eating a little something every few hours keeps my blood sugar more stable and prevents me from getting *too* hungry.

The Reboot Meal Plan

	BREAKFAST	SNACK	LUNCH	SNACK	DINNER
DAY 1	Green Basil Smoothie (page 107)	Chicken broth with Simple Wilted Greens (page 86)	Broiled Salmon and Fennel Salad (page 150)	Hard-boiled egg with either condiment (page 132)	Simple Salad of Bitter Greens (page 218), Amalfi Lemon Chicken (page 189)
DAY 2	Olive Oil–Scrambled Eggs with Arugula and Fennel Salad (page 115)	Celery Water (page 128)	Creamy Cauliflower Soup with Pepitas (page 134)	½ (7 ounces) leftover Green Basil Smoothie (from day 1)	Shrimp and Endive Salad (page 163), Millet Tabbouleh Salad (page 155)
DAY 3	Breakfast Chia Seed Pudding (page 111)	½ (7 ounces) leftover Green Basil Smoothie (from day 1)	White Bean and Broccoli Rabe Sauté (page 237), with chicken from batch cooking if you want	Celery Water (page 128)	Olive Oil–Poached Salmon (page 100), Simple Wilted Greens (page 86), ¼ cup quinoa (page 92)

HOW WILL I FEEL?

Everyone is going to react differently when the foods that have been hurting their gut are benched, and clean, nutrient-rich foods take their place. Some people feel amazing right away and find themselves full of energy, but if that's not you, don't worry. As your body starts to detox, you may feel a bit draggy or out of sorts. You might even find yourself feeling *more* bloated, or visiting the bathroom more often than usual, especially if you aren't used to eating a lot of high-fiber foods and greens. It's all par for the course, and these effects usually don't last more than a few days.

If your system is very sensitive, as mine is, you might have a more extreme reaction if you make a lot of changes all at once. If you have a powerful addiction to one of the foods you're avoiding during the reboot, the way I do to sugar, you might even have withdrawal symptoms, like headaches or flu-like aches. If that's the case, you may need to work your way up to a full reboot a little more gently, eliminating different food categories one at a time. Don't get discouraged! In some ways this is as much a fact-finding mission as anything, and you have just taken a big step toward identifying something that your body reacts to strongly. So take your time. You'll get there eventually. And when you do, *you're* the one who will be in control!

GET COMFORTABLE BEING A BIT HUNGRY NOW AND THEN

How often are you really, truly, unbearably hungry? The truth is we've trained ourselves to fear even the *idea* of hunger. Lots of times we eat before we reach that threshold just to avoid an anticipated discomfort. I'm so paranoid about letting my blood sugar get too low (and the crankies and headaches that come with it) that I often snack on the nuts or chocolate I've stashed in my bag even though I'm not really hungry. Other times we eat because we are dehydrated and actually just need some water. The next time you find yourself eating because the clock says you should, or because you might not get a chance later, or because everyone else is ordering food, think about how hungry you actually feel. Remember, in this as in all things, it's smart to follow your gut!

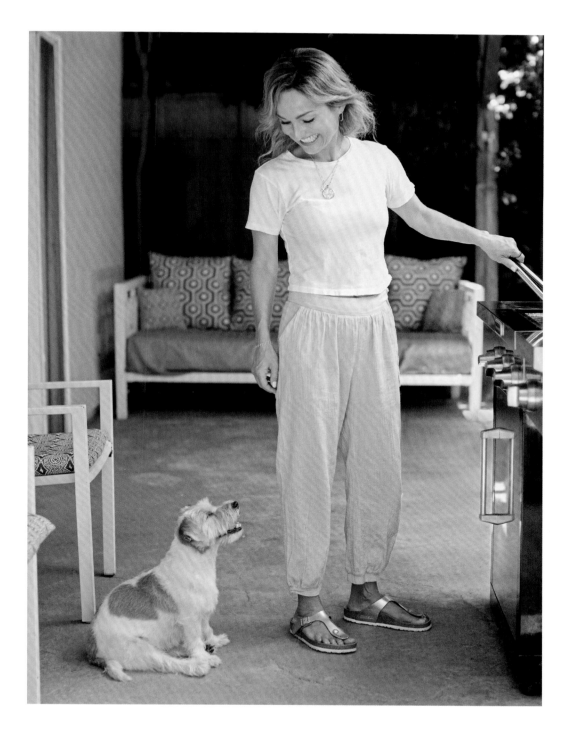

CHAPTER 7

Optimize Your Life: Taking It to the Next Level

Once I figured out a way of eating that worked for me, I was well on the road to recovery. But I couldn't really heal the damage that four decades of not-always-great choices had done to my body overnight. Nor could I necessarily get there through food alone. It all starts with food, but it became clear to me over time that I also needed to fine-tune other parts of my lifestyle to better support me and help the healing continue.

I am not suggesting you add all of these practices to your routine, or even any of them if the simple act of changing your diet helps you live your best life. As I've said, I'm convinced eating well is the single best thing you can do for your health. But if you're ready to expand your journey to wellness into other aspects of your lifestyle, you may want to check out some of the things I've found that amplify the effects of a healthy diet and keep me looking and feeling the way I want to.

This chapter includes an overview of the extra measures I've incorporated into my life to ensure that my body functions at the highest possible levels, my digestive system works efficiently, and the factors that caused me to get sick in the first place—an unbalanced diet, stress, and environmental toxins—don't ever get the upper hand again.

Now, I readily admit that I don't have the fear of doctors that many people do; to the contrary, both my mother and Jade routinely roll their eyes and call me a hypochondriac when I announce I'm off to the doctor (again . . .). But I know I wouldn't have reached the state of health I'm in now if I hadn't been willing to try some things that might raise a few eyebrows. And, not to be overly dramatic, but the experience of losing a beloved brother to cancer when he was only thirty has also made me painfully aware that ignoring warning signs, at any age, can have the most serious consequences imaginable. At the end of the day I'm a very pragmatic person, and I'm convinced that when there is a problem, the solution is out there if you are willing to do some research, form an opinion that's guided by the advice of smart people you trust, and keep at it until you've turned things around. That attitude has gotten me pretty far in life . . . so don't give up!

Even if you are not actively sick, routinely seeing your general practitioner, a nutritionist, a functional medicine doctor (one who looks at the whole body to find the root cause of disease), or an acupuncturist can help you achieve a state of wellness that may minimize or even prevent illness. As far as I'm concerned, it's always better to address the root cause of any discomfort than to treat only the symptoms, and establishing a trusting, open-ended relationship with your doctors is an essential part of staying healthy. Don't wait until you feel sick to schedule a visit!

Acupuncture

I've been getting acupuncture treatments for more than a decade now, and to me they are one of the pillars of my wellness routine. I see my long-time acupuncturist, Dr. Deborah Kim, who is also a master herbalist and holistic nutritionist, once a week when I can, and I really credit her with putting me on a better path to wellness.

I began seeing Debbie when I was starting to think about getting pregnant. I'd been taking birth control for years, and when my menstrual cycles still hadn't resumed a year after I went off the pill, my ob-gyn suggested I try acupuncture to reopen those pathways. It worked, and Debbie has been a trusted part of my health team ever since. Together, we have worked on stress modulation, immune strengthening, digestion, and relief of the pain I sometimes have in my jaw, neck, and back.

Muscle Testing and Supplements

I learned about muscle testing when my brother was sick, almost twenty years ago, and at that time the practice was considered pretty far out there. But I had done some research about the benefits of nutritional supplements for patients being treated for cancer and tracked down someone who used this form of biofeedback to diagnose nutritional deficiencies. Unfortunately, my brother thought it was crazy voodoo nonsense, but I was intrigued by the concept.

By the time I started working with my acupuncturist, the practice of muscle testing had become a lot more mainstream. Debbie uses a version known as Nutrition Response Testing, and it's another way she gets feedback about where there are weaknesses and deficiencies in the body. In this simple, noninvasive process, she applies pressure to my extended arm at the same time she places small jars with capsules of nutritional supplements on my abdomen. Some make my muscles better able to resist the pressure of her hand against mine, while others make me weaker. Based on the results of that muscle response, and anything I might have told her about how I'm feeling, she adjusts my regimen of supplements. I know it sounds strange, but I've seen and felt the difference myself—it's amazing how your body knows what it needs!

While the specific supplements I take change from month to month, they always include digestive packs with pre- and probiotics and other things to keep my gut ecosystem humming; immune enhancers, like eyebright and andrographis; and various adaptogens. Some herbal supplements, especially ashwagandha, Siberian ginseng, cordyceps, rhodiola, and Schisandra, help the body adapt to stress; for some people, ashwagandha even has a mild antianxiety effect. From time to time I've also taken bacopa to help with brain fog. If you are under a lot of stress or have what Debbie calls a "high performance" lifestyle (guilty), you might want to read up on the benefits of supplements or consult a nutritionist. I'm convinced that strategic use of supplements has kept me in a place where I can function the way I need to.

Functional and Integrative Practitioners

I owe my hormonal health to my integrative doctor, who was the first to connect my digestive issues to my chronic sinusitis and the wild hormonal swings that were becoming a real problem for me. Like functional medicine doctors, integrative practitioners are trained in Western medicine (meaning they have MDs), but they treat the whole body, not simply symptoms of illness. Many integrative doctors bring an additional background in Eastern medicine to their diagnostic and treatment regimens too. When I first went for treatment, I really felt my hormonal problems were getting the better of me. Not just cranky PMS kind of mood swings; for two weeks of the month I looked and felt like I was four months pregnant! It got to the point where the stylist for my Food Network show wanted to tear his hair out, because I was going up or down two full dress sizes in a matter of days—he couldn't keep up with me! All the travel, digestive

WHY DO I NEED SUPPLEMENTS IF I'M EATING SO WELL?

Even though I've made many positive adjustments to my diet, I still cover my bases with nutritional supplements. Dr. Debbie Kim explained their importance to me this way: "Our modern diets just don't provide the same kind of nutritional balance and variety they did fifty or a hundred years ago. For example, organ meats like liver, kidneys, and heart contain many nutrients our body needs, and they work hand in hand with the nutrients we get from muscle meat. But few people have a plate of liver for dinner anymore, while we overeat on steaks and pork chops. Without the balance of nutrients that you get from 'whole hog' eating—eating the entire animal, not just the prime cuts—you can become more prone to cancer. Not only that, as the monocropping practices of industrial farming reduce the number of different fruits and vegetables that make it to our tables every day, they are also limiting the kinds of nutrients we get from what we eat. So I think almost everyone can benefit from nutritional supplements.

"I'm not talking about mass-produced all-in-one supplements made from synthetic nutrients, though. I only recommend dietary supplements derived from plants and other foods. Our bodies know how to extract the nutrients from food; they have been doing it for centuries. The vitamin C you get from eating an orange is very different from ascorbic acid manufactured in a lab, which is literally one molecule away from the asphalt we use to make sidewalks! Plus, nature knows how to deliver nutrients most efficiently, and in real food they occur in combinations that make them more readily available to your body. You can actually take a lower dosage than you get in that one-a-day capsule because your body can access and use every bit.

"The good thing is these supplements come with very little baggage—you can't really overdose on broccoli! They also allow us to get the benefits of foods we don't usually eat in big quantities, like ginger or turmeric, more conveniently."

issues, sinus infections, lack of good sleep, and stress from long periods of work without any real time off, compounded by the natural process of aging, had put me in some serious hormonal distress.

Hormonal supplements helped to get me back on track, but my integrative doctor made it clear to me that lifestyle changes were also critical to regulating my hormones. As with so many health issues, you can medicate the symptoms, but ultimately it's getting to the heart of the problem—meaning taking positive steps toward better nutrition, exercise, and sleep—that will bring the greatest benefits. Check with your ob-gyn about getting your hormone levels checked if you have concerns, especially if you are nearing menopause, but don't end your journey there. It all works hand in hand.

Vitamin Push

From time to time, if I've been away from home a lot and not getting good sleep, or if I feel a cold coming on, I go to my functional doctor for a concentrated dose of immunity-boosting vitamins called an IV push. She makes me a customized IV "cocktail" based on my most recent blood work, so I address any deficiencies and don't get anything I don't need (which would generally just pass right through).

Ayurveda

This very ancient Indian practice is a natural approach to nourishing the mind, body, and spirit. It uses food, holistic medicines, and treatments to replenish, detoxify, and balance the body to prevent aging and disease. I was first exposed to ayurvedic medicine when a close friend was diagnosed with breast cancer, and she had supplemented her Western treatments with ayurvedic ones to help keep things in balance. I was intrigued and decided to accompany her on a retreat. Since then I try to make time for a three- to five-day retreat once every year or so.

These retreats are pretty rigorous affairs; we eat no meat, dairy, fish, or gluten—just rice and legumes, dals, and lots and lots of vegetables. Every day there are different treatments meant to help eliminate accumulated toxins, including four-handed massages, scrubs, vagina steams, visits to a sweat lodge, and more, all tailored to rebalancing the five basic elements that make up our bodies: earth, water, fire, wind, and space (I'm most ruled by wind and fire— no surprise for a fiery Italian!).

Retreats are not cheap (although there are certainly high-end spas that can set you back five times what my favorite ayurvedic center costs), but it's hard to put a price on how hydrated, unblocked, and at peace I feel after these visits. Sometimes, especially if I'm shooting a Food Network show and won't have time to prepare meals for myself,

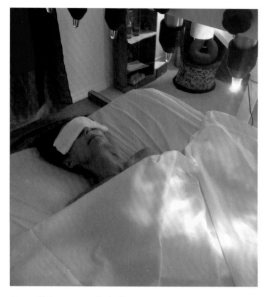

A purifying crystal chakra treatment was part of my Panchakarma ayurvedic retreat.

I have ayurvedic meals delivered and eat one per day, usually for lunch, five days a week. I've become so addicted to the chef's ayurvedic Kale Pesto that he's given me permission to include it in this book (see page 89)!

There are numerous companies that can administer intravenous supplements, either in a commercial setting or even in your home, but in my opinion you should consult with your doctor before pursuing this option. He or she may offer this treatment at the office, or have guidance on which specific nutrients are most appropriate and beneficial for your personal health concerns

Meditation

I wish I could say I start and end every day with thirty minutes of absolute stillness, finding time amid the chaos to quiet my brain and let all the tensions of the day recede as I sit cross-legged on my perfect meditation pillow. That's the goal, and I envy those who have learned to achieve it, but I'm not quite there yet. I'm working on it!

I *have* found that even five or ten minutes of deep relaxation right before bed has a valuable soothing, calming effect on me, and I've become pretty good about carving out at least that much time for a form of meditation every day. Rather than sitting cross-legged, I prefer to lie on the floor with my knees bent and my feet flat on the floor, making as much contact with the unpadded surface as possible, and my hands at my sides, palms up. In this position I breathe in and out as deeply as possible, filling not only my chest but my belly, too, and expelling each breath as fully as I can. Focusing on this breathing helps me short-circuit that loop in my brain replaying the day's events over and over and lets me unwind from the stress of the day—or, if I do it in the morning, it puts me in a good frame of mind for going out to face the world.

Detoxes

It goes without saying that the best way to detox is to avoid consuming toxins in the first place, but that's easier said than done. Toxins in the environment, in the cleaning products we use on our bodies and in our homes, even in the clothing we wear, can all find their way into our systems, especially if you have vulnerabilities. For me, it was my sinuses, which always seemed to be the weak link in my immune defenses, and my digestive system.

Our liver, kidneys, and digestive system do the lion's share of filtering out these toxins, so whenever I can, I like to give them an assist. These are a few of my favorite detox practices:

Water filters: Los Angeles is famous for having water that looks and tastes funky, but in many parts of the country what comes out of the tap can have contaminants such as heavy metals and chemicals, at levels ranging from not great to downright alarming. While they can't remove everything, water filters will strain out some of the nasties in your cooking and drinking water. If you have concerns about the water quality in your area, invest in a water pitcher with a built-in filter or, better yet, attach a filter to the cold water tap in your kitchen to ensure you are using filtered water for all your food preparation.

Korean scrubs: My aunt Raffy was the first to get me hooked on these treatments, and we try to make a trip to our favorite Korean spa at least once a year. The process is both refreshingly low tech and not for the modest: your aesthetician will essentially scour every inch of your naked body with two rough-textured mitts until the dry, dead skin rolls off like sand after a day at the beach. But afterward you will feel unbelievably smooth, soft, and hydrated, and the price tag is usually quite reasonable.

Air purifiers: I'm a big fan of air purifiers and have them throughout my house to capture airborne bacteria, dust, and other pollutants. I've found they really help me in my battle against sinus infections. If you have seasonal allergies or other sensitivities, or live in an area where air pollution is a problem—and sadly, that is all too many of us—an air purifier is a smart investment. Be vigilant about washing or replacing the filters as directed, and you will find the purifiers make a big difference in the air quality at home.

Flannel and castor oil packs: It was actually my daughter's sitter who introduced me to this treatment, and I admit I was skeptical the first time I tried it. But I'd been complaining about my stomach problems, and she suggested this old folk remedy; I figured why not give it a try. To my surprise, it had a seriously strong detoxifying effect! The process was messy but pretty simple: I saturated a piece of flannel (you can buy these at most health food stores specifically for this purpose) with castor oil and placed it on my abdomen, topping it with a warm heating pad or hot water bottle. (It's a good idea to wrap the heating pad in a plastic bag to keep it clean.)

Keep it on for 45 to 60 minutes. The heat helps intensify the detoxifying effect of the castor oil, and many feel it helps with circulation, inflammation, and pain from menstrual symptoms. And it sure beats taking the oil by the spoonful! I do this once or twice a year.

Infrared Sauna

Unlike traditional saunas, which heat the room around you, infrared saunas heat you from *within*, releasing toxins and helping you to eliminate them through your skin. Not only is this a lot less stifling than a regular sauna, it's actually quite relaxing, as you lie on a bed inside a pod-like machine throughout the treatment. Many people report that their skin looks amazing afterward, and you can even burn off a bunch of calories! To help the toxins drain even more efficiently, before an infrared treatment I put on a compression suit for twenty minutes. This gets the stagnant fluids in my systems moving so I can sweat them out.

Sleep

This should be the easiest one, right? After all, sleep is a natural as breathing. But somehow we never seem to prioritize rest, or even set aside enough hours in

COFFEE AND SUGAR BODY SCRUB

½ cup medium-grind coffee

¾ cup turbinado sugar, preferably organic

¼ cup kosher salt

½ cup olive oil (no need to use expensive extra-virgin oil)

Not up for the quasi-exhibitionist experience of a spa scrub-down? You can get similar effects in your own bathroom. I like to do it after a workout, before I shower. Start by combining the ingredients at left and applying the scrub mixture on your skin while it's still dry. Rub firmly with a dry washcloth or mesh scrubbing mitt, or use a dry brush to exfoliate every inch you can reach (excluding your face and eye area). Rinse off any remnants, shower as usual, and then moisturize generously!

the day for a full night's sleep. I know I've been guilty of that more times than I can count, especially since becoming a mom and traveling more for work. It just seems there's always so much to do, right?

But sleeping is not the same as doing nothing; in fact, a whole lot goes on while we sleep, and it has been proven that lack of sleep can actually *cause* inflammation. Sleep is the time when our cells regroup and regenerate, a process that simply can't happen when we are awake and using all of our bodily resources. When you are deprived of sleep, your body reacts as it would to an illness, generating a complicated chain of responses that triggers an immune response.

I've learned I can't just leave sleep to chance if I want to function well, so now I help it along. My mini-meditation practice lets me chill out so I can ease into sleep more quickly, and I've also started taking supplements of magnesium, calcium lactate, and Min-Tran (a mineral complex) before bed to help calm the central nervous system and relax my muscles. These let me sleep more deeply and with fewer interruptions. There are also calming drinks made with magnesium that many people (including my mother and sister) find help them get better rest.

Exercise/Yoga

I've heard diet, exercise, and sleep described as the three-legged stool of health, but for a lot of years, this leg was a little wobbly for me. With travel and an unpredictable work schedule, I really wasn't able to carve out regular gym time, and even though I love outdoor sports, the occasional (read: infrequent) bike ride or walk on the beach just wasn't cutting it.

When I was pregnant with Jade, my obstetrician suggested I try yoga, and I've been a huge convert ever since. The combination of calming breathwork and strength-building stretches genuinely

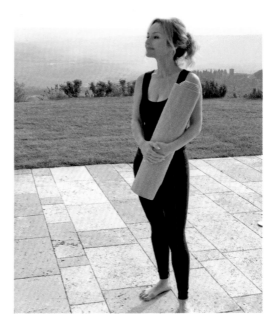

reshaped my body. And I found the concentration required to perfect the poses and move through the sequences helped me shut out the noise in a way that taking a spin class never had. It's not an exaggeration to say that yoga changed my whole attitude toward exercise, and I do some kind of yoga, even if it's just a few stretches, every single day, whether I'm home or traveling.

Lately, I've been mixing up my regular vinyasa workouts with Yin Yoga, a gentler practice that uses seated and reclining poses that are held for longer periods of time to help release the spine, hips, and pelvis. It's incredibly soothing. I've also begun taking a Pilates class here and there to help with my posture and muscle strength.

The point is not that yoga is the "perfect" exercise, or that it's right for everyone just because it's right for me. If exercise isn't already a part of your life, you may need to experiment with a few different workouts or activities before you find something that really speaks to you. You don't have to go to a gym or a classroom; there are tons of streaming programs and YouTube teachers that bring instruction to you at home. Or get a dog and commit to walking her ten thousand steps a day. The important thing is to keep trying until you find something that you can commit to, because without some kind of regular movement in your life, sooner or later that stool is going to tip over!

Reboot

I like to reboot my digestive system two or three times a year with a superstrict cleansing diet. I'm most likely to do this right after a vacation or the holidays—times when I'm doing less home cooking or attending more social events, and eating less well than I should. I find a quick reboot is like a jolt to the system in a good way, and it reminds me how much better I feel when I give my gut the things it likes best. For the specifics of my three-day reboot, see chapter 6.

Intermittent Fasting

Think about how you feel when you work through a weekend or go too long without a vacation. In a way, your gut is the same. When it's working its hardest to handle every new thing you're sending its way before it's had the chance to digest and dispose of what was already there, it doesn't know what to attack first. Things slip through the cracks, and the small irritants and inflammations that your very efficient digestive system can usually deal with easily are allowed to rage unnoticed— until you can't *help* but notice. Fasting is a way to give your gut a chance to clean out its inbox and marshal its energies before you start assigning it new tasks.

DETOX TEA

½ cup peeled and roughly chopped ginger root

2 tablespoons peeled and roughly chopped turmeric root (optional)

Zest of 1 lemon, removed with a vegetable peeler

2 tablespoons fresh lemon juice, from 1 lemon

When I'm doing a reboot (see page 57) and trying to limit my caffeine intake, I substitute a cup of this warm, spicy tea for my midmorning or afternoon Americano break. If you're not detoxing, feel free to add a drizzle of honey, but I find it delicious as is.

Combine the ginger, turmeric (if using), lemon zest, and lemon juice in a saucepan with 6 cups water and simmer for 10 minutes. Let the tea steep for 5 minutes off the heat, then strain and serve or refrigerate for up to 3 days and reheat before serving.

There are different ways to approach fasting, including true fasting—abstaining from any food other than clear liquids for twenty-four hours or more—and intermittent fasting, which many people find a lot more manageable. Intermittent fasting means you confine all your meals to a set period of time, usually eight hours, and don't eat outside of that period at all. This gives your body a good long stretch without food so it can repair and restore itself.

I find sixteen hours is a long time to go without eating, even if much of that time is spent sleeping. Doctors I've spoken to say you can get the same benefit from a shorter fast of fourteen or even twelve

hours—especially if you do a true fast day every now and then. Whichever feels comfortable and achievable to you is fine; the important thing is to give your gut some downtime. And if you're like me and sometimes find it's already noon before you've thought about making yourself something to eat, this might be a good strategy for you!

As my mind opens and I start to understand my body more and more, I realize keeping my bucket of toxins at a manageable level and not approaching that tipping point into sickness isn't something I can do alone. It takes a village. So talk to your health-care providers, listen to podcasts and read books, talk to your friends and encourage one another, dip your toe into a new workout, resolve to make sleep a bigger priority in your life. Every little step will get you further along your own journey.

Most important, remember that these are long-term solutions, not "miracle" cures. It's not like popping an aspirin for a headache and getting instant results; you're addressing the underlying causes of health problems that have taken years to develop. You will get there in time, and I'm going to make sure you are well fed every step of the way. Now on to the recipes!

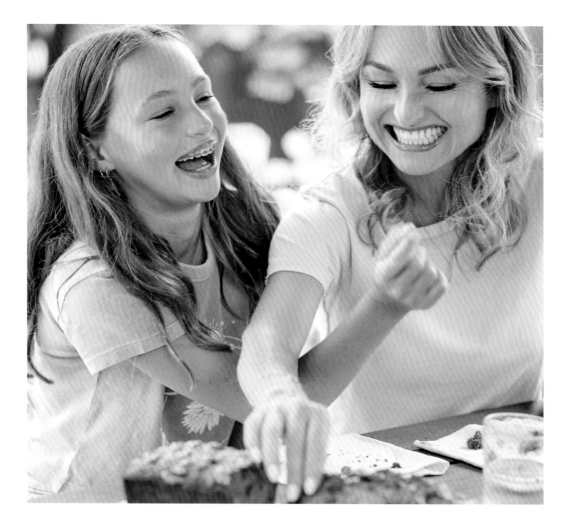

PART II

THE RECIPES

Let the Healing Begin

Welcome to the main event: the recipes! These are the dishes that I've used—and still use—to make a real change in the way my gut works and my body feels. I created them specifically to reduce stress on my digestive system and support my immune health while maximizing the flavors, textures, and colors that keep me coming back for seconds. I feel confident they can do the same for you.

In these recipes I've used foods associated with inflammation sparingly, or even sidestepped them entirely if I found an alternative that gave me a result that was still beautiful, tasted amazing, and felt celebratory. When I do dip into Proceed with Caution (see page 23), I make every delicious bite count and do my best to make smart changes that help mitigate their impact on my system. While sticking primarily to my modern Italian playbook, I have made a few side trips into the flavor palates of other international cuisines to keep things interesting, simple, and tasty, especially in the "Lean and Clean" chapter (page 126), which features recipes free of all dairy, wheat, and nightshades (read: no pasta, Parmesan, or tomatoes!).

My goal was to create a sensual experience around "healthy food." As always, I use generous amounts of citrus to add brightness; nuts, toasted grains, or shards of crunchy Parm to add texture; and big handfuls of fresh herbs to make my dishes a little lighter and brighter. Sensory impressions are key here too—they kick in long before you put the food in your mouth and create anticipation. I'm thinking of the scent of fresh basil or rosemary and how it not only perfumes the air while you're cooking or chopping, but also sends a signal to your brain that something good is coming. Your eyes take in the vibrant colors of fresh produce, or the gorgeous crisped skin of a roasted chicken breast that you've sliced and drizzled with lemony pan juices—you can practically taste it before, well, tasting it! The sensual and experiential part of cooking is something I love, and it's an integral part of the romanticism of Italian food.

In the chapters that follow you'll find my new favorite breakfasts, lunches, and dinners, plus a few more-indulgent recipes for sweet treats. There's also a selection of recipes that are extra lean and clean, including snack options that will be kinder to your system than anything you can get from a vending machine (or a drive-through!). If you're someone who likes to have all your ducks in a row at the beginning of the week, you're going to love the chapter on batch cooking, which will help you prep and strategize for no-cook or minimal-cook meals when time and inspiration are in short supply.

However you use these recipes, I hope you find every one of them flavorful, easy to prepare, and truly nourishing in every sense of the word.

CHAPTER 8

Batch It Up!

If you're looking to make real changes to the way you eat, making home-cooked food is a huge step in the right direction. Obviously, it's easier to control what goes into your mouth if you only eat food you've made yourself. On the other hand, all that cooking takes time, and I don't know too many people who are up for cooking three meals from scratch day in and day out—even me!

The recipes in this chapter are your shortcut to eating healthy, wholesome, home-cooked food without spending your life in the kitchen. With a selection of these easily made building blocks at the ready, you can assemble, rather than cook, meals that are kind to your gut yet take next to no time at all to put together. Combine two, three, or more for an easy, breezy lunch or dinner—or even breakfast if that's how you roll.

Recipes with a (RB) symbol are compatible with the reboot cleanse on page 57.

MIXING AND MATCHING YOUR WAY TO RECIPE-FREE MEALS

The key is having a few simple, storage-friendly precooked components on hand at all times so you can quickly improvise a fast soup, salad, or grain bowl when mealtime rolls around (see IMPROV meals on page 50). All the recipes in this chapter yield relatively large amounts and keep well in the fridge for at least three days. With a few of these ingredients ready to go, it is truly effortless to improvise a simple yet satisfying meal in under five minutes.

Think of these recipes as foundation ingredients that you can either combine or supplement with fresh greens, leftover cooked veggies, or protein from last night's dinner. If you have some kind of grain (millet, brown rice, quinoa) and some cooked protein (hard-boiled eggs, bits of cooked chicken, beans), all you need are veggies and more veggies to make something nourishing and sustaining without ever having to hunt down a recipe or consult a meal plan. Feel free to liven things up with any of the "superfoods" on page 38 to add texture and brightness, and check out chapter 14, "The Side Hustle," for a dozen more dishes that are perfect partners to mix and match.

Here are some ideas:

* Start with a bowl of raw greens and top with ¼ cup cooked grains or beans and cooked veggies of any kind. Ladle on hot broth.

* Make a breakfast bowl with ½ cup cooked rice or quinoa, quartered eggs, and a little pile of cooked greens. Drizzle with a bit of evoo and a sprinkle of flake salt.

* Toss a couple handfuls of baby arugula or spring mix with a tablespoon or two of cooked grains and top with strips of Lemon and Oregano Pounded Chicken (page 99). Spoon a bit of Kale Pesto (page 89) over all.

* Arrange cooked greens and ¼ cup cooked beans in a bowl; pour hot broth over all and sprinkle on a bit of grated pecorino.

* Pile chicken strips and roasted veggies on dressed greens. Add a few olives and chopped nuts.

* Mix sautéed greens or roasted veggies into beaten eggs for a fast frittata.

* Pair some of last night's leftover broiled salmon or steak salad with lightly dressed lentils and sautéed greens.

These are just a few of the possibilities; I'm sure you will come up with your own favorites. The point is to have clean, healthy, and satisfying food ready to go at the drop of a hat. Think outside the box about what constitutes a meal, and focus on assembling a variety of textures, colors, and flavors. Before you know it, you might start to wonder why you ever needed a recipe in the first place.

It may feel like a lot of work the first time you try this approach, but once you see how much time a single prep session saves over the course of the week, you'll quickly come to think of it as a great investment in your health.

WEEKEND GAME PLAN

I find the weekend is a great time to stock my fridge with a few easy meal components, whether for IMPROV meals (page 50) or for making weeknight cooking a little faster. I like to prep and cook over the course of an afternoon—I often multitask, using the time while I'm cooking to catch up on podcasts or have a nice long check-in phone call with my mother in Italy!

The specific items to make are up to you, but I always like to have a couple quarts of chicken broth (for soups, risottos, or sauces), at least one cooked grain and/or legume, some roasted or sautéed veggies (or both), and one cooked protein.

If you are a multicooker fan, you can put it to good use here, especially for long-cooked

things like broth and dried beans. But even using conventional stovetop methods, this kind of meal prep isn't that time consuming. Start by putting a chicken on for broth, removing and setting aside the cooked meat after it has simmered for an hour. In that time you'll have been able to poach or roast a couple of salmon fillets, roast a sheet pan of chopped veggies, and cook a pot of brown rice or quinoa. While your grains cook, wash and sauté a mess of greens (I'm partial to Swiss chard these days, but whatever you prefer is A-OK) and hard-boil a half-dozen eggs. Let everything cool, then pack it all up in covered containers; you might even want to freeze some if you've made really big batches of grains, proteins, or broth to get a head start on the next week.

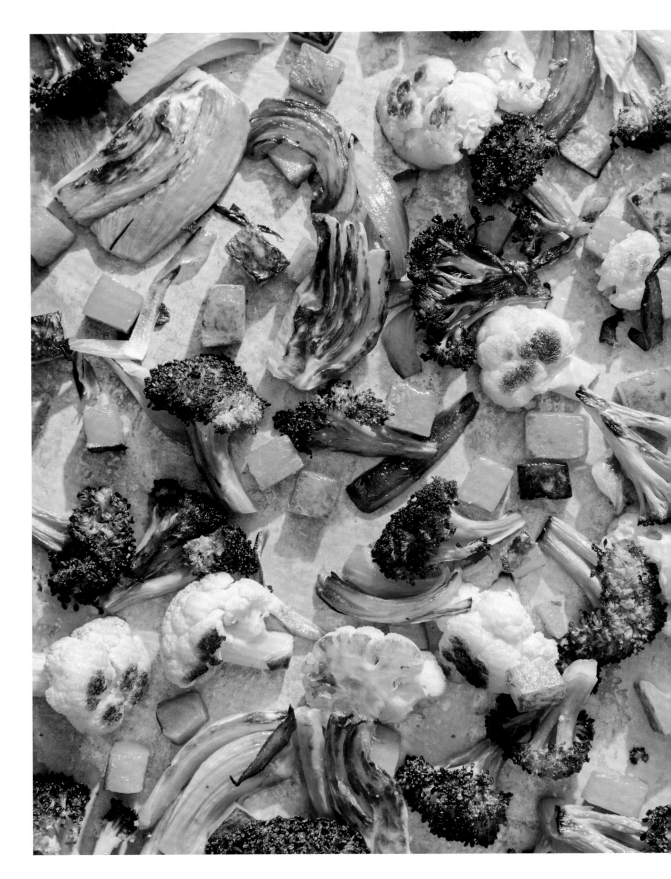

BIG BATCH ROASTED VEGGIES

SERVES 6 TO 8

I've found that Jade—and most kids—love vegetables when they have been roasted. Roasting concentrates the flavors and caramelizes the sugars in vegetables like broccoli, making them taste a bit sweeter. The crispier they are, the more she'll eat! I make this at least three times a week. Don't waste the broccoli stems; sometimes I peel and slice them to roast along with the florets; other times I just save them for crudités or grate them for a slaw.

1 head of broccoli, cut into large florets

1 head of cauliflower, cut into large florets

1 half butternut squash, peeled, seeds removed, and cut into ½-inch dice

1 fennel bulb, stalks removed, bulb cut into ⅓-inch wedges

1 red onion, cut into ⅓-inch wedges

¼ cup olive oil

1 tablespoon kosher salt

Preheat the oven to 450°F.

Place the broccoli, cauliflower, squash, fennel, and onion in a large bowl. Drizzle with the oil, season with salt, and toss well to coat. Divide the vegetables between two rimmed baking sheets.

Roast the vegetables for about 20 minutes, or until they start to brown. Stir the vegetables, rotate the baking sheets back to front and top rack to bottom, and roast for 10 minutes longer, or until tender. To store, refrigerate the cooled veggies in a covered container for up to 5 days.

BAKED CORIANDER
SWEET POTATOES

SERVES 2 TO 4

Sweet potatoes are so dense and hearty, I often make them the center-piece of a meatless meal. Served with a salad or some sautéed greens, this is a filling but nearly effortless lunch or dinner; as a side, half a potato is an ample portion.

2 sweet potatoes, scrubbed but not peeled

1 tablespoon olive oil, plus ¼ cup to finish

2 teaspoons coriander seeds, toasted and cracked

1 teaspoon grated lemon zest

1 teaspoon flake salt

1 tablespoon roughly chopped fresh flat-leaf parsley leaves (optional)

Preheat the oven to 425 F.

Place the sweet potatoes on a rimmed baking sheet. Pierce each potato a few times with the tip of a knife and rub with 1 tablespoon olive oil. Roast until the potatoes are soft all the way through, about 1 hour, turning them halfway through cooking. Set aside to cool for 5 minutes.

Cut the potatoes in half and fluff the insides with a fork. Drizzle each half with a tablespoon of olive oil and sprinkle with a few coriander seeds, some lemon zest, and flake salt.

Top with parsley, if desired.

BASIC BROCCOLI RABE

SERVES 4

Blanched broccoli rabe holds up well in the refrigerator for up to 5 days, making it a great choice for prep day. Add it to pastas or grain bowls, or serve it as a side dish topped with something savory like the Roasted Garlic Dressing on page 220.

1 bunch of broccoli rabe, tough ends trimmed

2 tablespoons extra-virgin olive oil

½ teaspoon flake salt

Crushed red pepper flakes, grated lemon zest, or grated Parmigiano-Reggiano (optional), for garnish

Bring a large pot of water to a boil over high heat. Season well with kosher salt.

Add the broccoli rabe to the boiling water and cook for 3 minutes, or until the stems are just tender when pierced with a fork. Use tongs or a skimmer to transfer the rabe to a rimmed baking sheet to cool slightly.

When cool enough to handle, squeeze gently to remove as much liquid as possible. To serve, scatter on a platter and drizzle with the olive oil. Top with a sprinkle of flake salt and the garnish of your choice, if desired. Serve warm or at room temperature.

To store, refrigerate in a covered container for up to 5 days.

SIMPLE WILTED GREENS

SERVES 4 TO 6

If I'm not having a salad with my meal, a serving of cooked greens is my fall-back to ensure I'm getting some of their essential prebiotics every day. This recipe will work with any kind of greens, from hardy ones like kale to the most tender, like spinach, in whatever proportions you like. The cooked greens will keep up to three days in the fridge, and are so convenient to toss into a grain bowl with some lentils and roasted veggies, or fold into an omelet. If I'm entertaining, I might reheat them in a sauté pan with some slivers of sun-dried tomatoes or olives to jazz them up.

2½ tablespoons olive oil

1 garlic clove, smashed and peeled

1 shallot, chopped

1½ teaspoons kosher salt

2 pounds mixed hardy, medium-tender, and tender greens, such as Tuscan kale, escarole, and spinach (see Note), chopped

Heat a large straight-sided skillet over medium-high heat. Add the oil and heat for another minute. Add the garlic and shallot and season with ¼ teaspoon of the salt. Cook, stirring often, for 2 minutes, or until the shallot is soft and fragrant. Add the greens to the pan and stir to coat in the oil. Reduce the heat slightly to medium and cover the pan. Steam for 4 minutes.

Uncover the pan and stir in the escarole and ¾ teaspoon of the salt. Cover the pan once again and steam for 2 minutes. Uncover the pan and add the spinach and the remaining ½ teaspoon salt. Increase the heat to medium-high and cook, stirring and tossing often, until the spinach is just wilted, about 1 minute. Serve hot.

NOTE ─────────────

Use the guide to substitute whichever greens you prefer or have on hand and adjust the total cooking time to reflect the hardiest vegetable; if you use only medium-tender and tender greens, for example, the greens should steam for only 2 minutes before adding the most tender ones, or about 3 minutes total.

HARDY GREENS: Tuscan kale, curly kale, red kale, savoy or green cabbage

─────────────

MEDIUM-TENDER GREENS: escarole; collards; mustard, beet, or turnip greens; dandelion greens, Swiss chard, bok choy

─────────────

TENDER GREENS: baby kale, arugula, watercress, pea shoot leaves

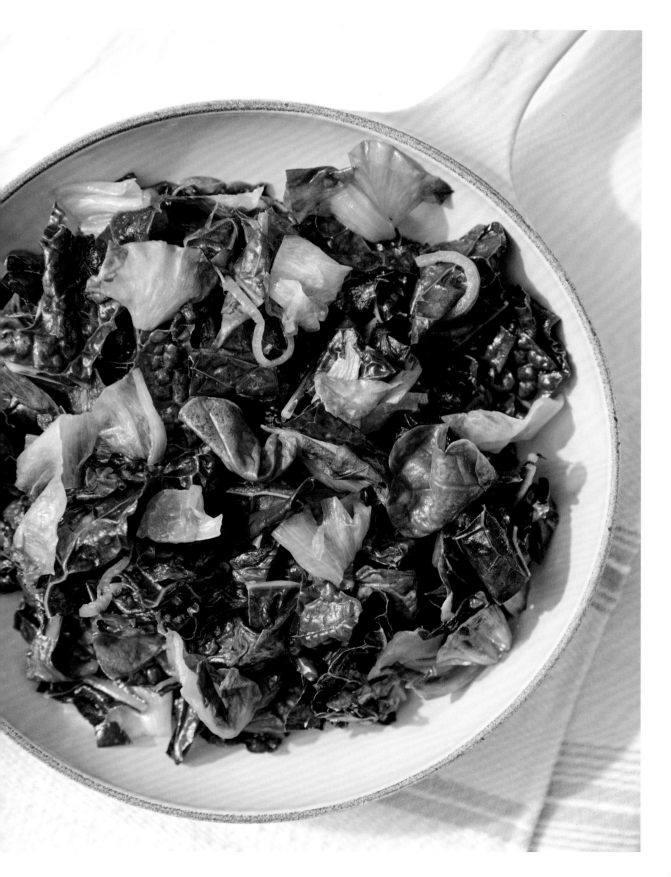

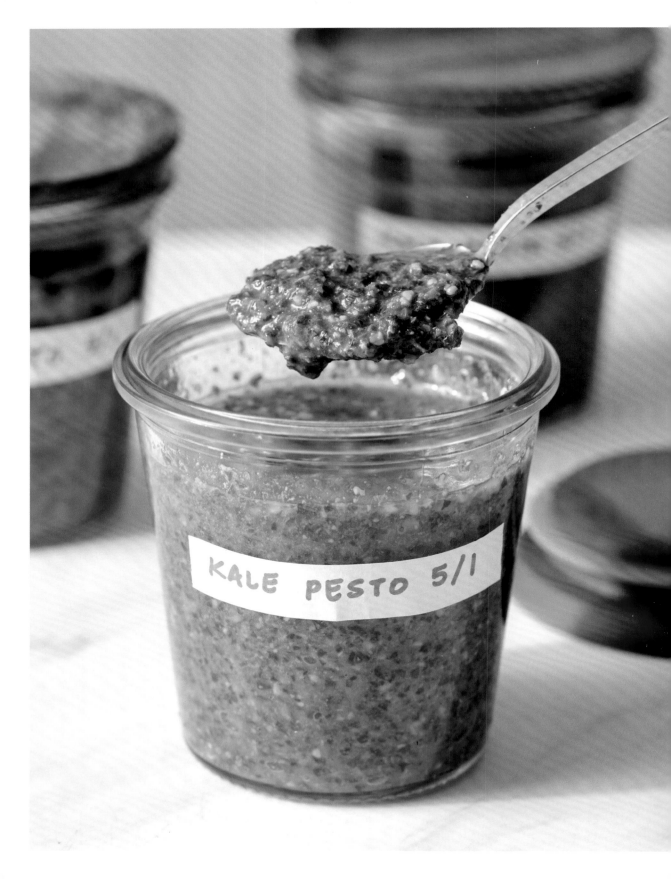

KALE PESTO

MAKES ABOUT 2 CUPS

Now and then I treat myself to meal deliveries from a local ayurvedic caterer who goes by the name of Chef Om. This all-purpose green sauce is based on one he makes, and I would probably eat a slab of Styrofoam if it had a little of this drizzled on top—I love it that much. Plus, it's vegan, superfast to make, and good on anything from eggs to grains to broiled fish or chicken. Walnuts have an anti-inflammatory effect, and while the pesto isn't traditional, since there isn't any Parmigiano-Reggiano or pine nuts, it's still super satisfying.

⅓ cup walnuts

1 (5-ounce) container
    baby kale

½ cup extra-virgin olive oil

½ teaspoon grated
    lime zest

2 teaspoons fresh
    lime juice

1 teaspoon kosher salt

Pulse the walnuts in a food processor a few times until just coarsely chopped. Add the kale and pulse a few more times to break up the leaves a bit. Add the oil, lime zest and juice, and salt and puree until smooth.

Store the pesto in the refrigerator with a piece of plastic wrap pressed directly onto the surface to prevent it from discoloring. Use the pesto within 5 days.

(RB)

DRIED BEANS, ITALIAN-STYLE

MAKES ABOUT 6 CUPS

We ate quite a lot of beans when I was a kid, and when cooked this way, as my mom always made them, they taste like home to me. Use this method for any type of beans you like, checking them for doneness after 50 minutes. The beans can soak for up to 48 hours but no longer, or they will start to ferment. Cooked beans can be frozen for up to a month, but their texture will be less firm when defrosted, better for using in soups or stews.

2 cups dried cannellini (white) or cranberry beans

1 fresh rosemary sprig

1 dried bay leaf

3 garlic cloves, smashed and peeled

3 tablespoons olive oil

1 teaspoon kosher salt

Place the beans in a large pot with 6 cups water. Refrigerate and soak for 12 hours or overnight.

The next day, drain the soaked beans and rinse well. Transfer the beans to a heavy pot or Dutch oven and add the rosemary, bay leaf, garlic, and olive oil. Pour 5 cups water over the beans and bring to a simmer over medium heat. Reduce the heat to maintain a gentle simmer. Cook for 1 hour, stirring occasionally, or until the beans are just soft. Season with the salt, remove from the heat, and allow to sit for 30 minutes.

If not using the beans right away, refrigerate them in their cooking liquid in a covered container for up to 5 days.

A LOTTA LENTILS

MAKES ABOUT 5 CUPS

Lentils are a little easier to digest than other kinds of legumes, at least for me, and are incredibly versatile as a building block. They are also quick to make because they don't need soaking. I almost always have some cooked lentils on hand to use as a bed for fish or meat, to mix with broth and veggies for a superfast soup, or to stand in for meat in a salad. Green-ish French lentils and tiny black beluga lentils hold their shape best; brown lentils break down to a soft, saucy texture.

2 cups brown, French (Le Puy), or beluga lentils, rinsed

3 fresh thyme sprigs

1 garlic clove, smashed and peeled

1 teaspoon kosher salt

Combine the lentils in a saucepan with the thyme, garlic, and water to cover by 2 inches. Bring to a boil, then reduce the heat, stir in the salt, and simmer for 15 to 20 minutes, depending on the variety; start to check for tenderness after about 12 minutes. Brown lentils cook the quickest and will become mushy if overdone; other varieties take longer but will still be semifirm when cooked. Just keep checking.

When tender, drain the lentils, discarding the garlic and thyme, and allow to cool. Transfer to a covered container and refrigerate for up to 5 days.

BIG BATCH QUINOA

MAKES ABOUT 5 CUPS

I started eating quinoa more than a decade ago on a visit to Peru; it was new to me at that time and I fell hard for its nutty flavor—and also how easy it was to digest. Now I nearly always have a cooked batch in the fridge. It's perfect for stirring into soups, tossing with salads, and using as a bed for anything you might serve with couscous or rice. Plus, it doesn't get sticky or clumpy when stored. If you haven't used it all within a few days, no worries—it also freezes beautifully. All quinoa, regardless of color, tastes about the same, so choose whichever you prefer. I often opt for the pale tan quinoa because it looks like brown rice or couscous, and Jade is more likely to eat it if it looks familiar. In my experience the multicolor blends tend to cook unevenly, so stick to one color at a time.

2 cups tan, red, or black quinoa, rinsed

½ teaspoon kosher salt

Place the quinoa, salt, and 4 cups water in a medium saucepan. Set over medium heat and bring to a boil, then cover and reduce the heat to maintain a simmer. Simmer for 10 minutes, or until all the liquid is absorbed and the quinoa is plumped. Remove from the heat and allow to steam with the lid on for 10 minutes before fluffing with a fork.

Cool, then transfer to covered containers and store in the refrigerator for up to 5 days or freeze for up to 3 months.

FREEZING GRAINS

Nearly all grains freeze well and reheat quickly with little loss of flavor or texture. To store them neatly and make it easier to defrost small portions at a time, scoop the cooled grain into a zip-top freezer bag and lay the bag flat on the counter. Press the grains into a thin, flat layer, filling the bag evenly, then seal, pressing out as much air as possible. Place on a small baking sheet and freeze until solid. Store until ready to use, then break off just as much as you need, returning the rest of the frozen grain sheet to the freezer.

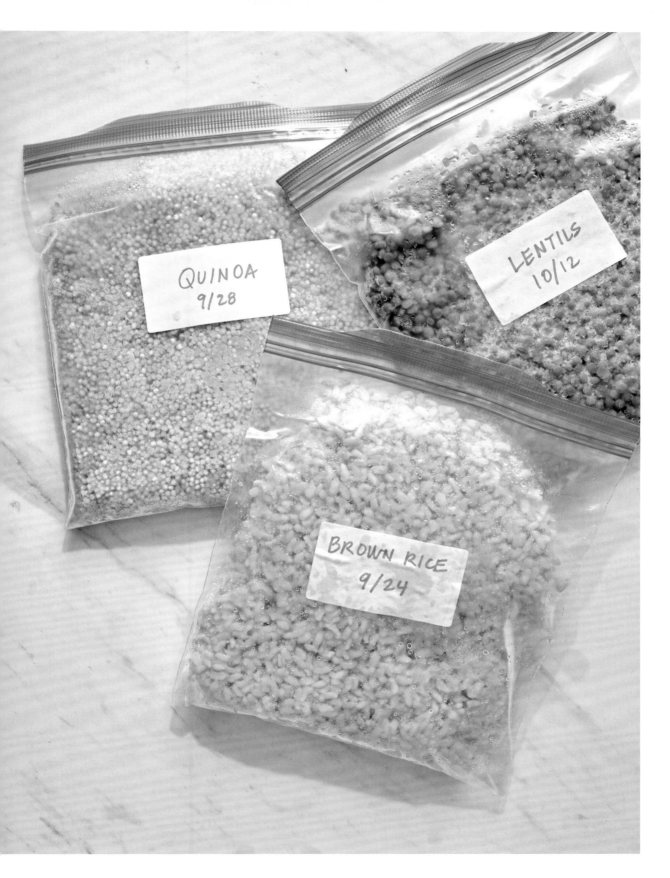

BIG BATCH BROWN RICE

MAKES ABOUT 6 CUPS

Because brown rice still has its hard bran covering, it takes about twice as long as white rice to cook, regardless of the variety. I like to make it in large batches and stash some in the freezer for quick meals. I like short-grain rice because it cooks up starchy, almost like a risotto, and I love basmati for its delicate perfume, but any brown rice will work in the recipes in this book. It freezes surprisingly well (see tips on page 92), and in fact the texture is even better for adding to stir-fries or grain salads after freezing.

2 cups brown rice
¾ teaspoon kosher salt

Place the rice in a fine-mesh strainer and rinse under running water; drain. Place the rinsed rice in a medium saucepan. Add the salt and 4 cups water and bring to a boil over medium heat. Reduce the heat to maintain a simmer. Cover and cook for 30 minutes, or until the rice is tender all the way through. Remove from the heat but leave covered for an additional 10 minutes to steam. Fluff with a fork.

Cool before transferring to covered containers. Refrigerate for up to 5 days or freeze for up to 3 months.

VEGETABLE BROTH

MAKES ABOUT 7 CUPS

Most of the commercial vegetable stocks on the shelves taste too strongly of onion and celery for my taste, so I prefer to make my own. It doesn't take nearly as long to make as chicken or meat stock, and it's a good way to use up produce that is not long for this world. This recipe is really a template, and you should tweak it to reflect your own palate and the state of your crisper. The only essential step is browning the onion really well—it adds a ton of flavor. After that, you're the boss!

½ onion

2 tomatoes, halved

4 garlic cloves, smashed and peeled

2 celery stalks, cut into thirds

2 carrots, cut into thirds

½ fennel bulb, tops and all, cut into 4 wedges

15 fresh thyme sprigs

8 fresh flat-leaf parsley sprigs

1 bay leaf

½ teaspoon whole black peppercorns

Heat a medium pot over medium heat. Place the onion and tomatoes cut side down on the bottom of the dry, hot pan. Cook for about 5 minutes, or until the onion is deep golden brown.

Add the garlic, celery, carrots, fennel, thyme, parsley, bay leaf, peppercorns, and 2 quarts water. Bring to a simmer over medium-high heat. Skim the broth, discarding any impurities that rise to the surface. Adjust the heat to maintain a gentle simmer and cook the broth, uncovered, for 1 hour. Remove from the heat and allow the broth to cool slightly for about 30 minutes. Strain through a fine-mesh strainer and cool completely. Store in the refrigerator for up to 5 days or freeze for up to 6 months.

TWO-FER CHICKEN BROTH

MAKES ABOUT 3 QUARTS BROTH AND 4 CUPS SHREDDED MEAT

One of the best examples I know of cooking smarter is this recipe, which yields lots of delicious, additive-free homemade broth, plus enough shredded cooked chicken meat for multiple lunches or dinners. Don't be tempted to substitute chicken pieces for the whole bird; the meat is much less likely to overcook when the bird is intact, and even when you pull off all the choice bits for another use, the carcass will continue to add flavor to the broth. Make a batch the next time you plan to be around the house for a few hours, and you will use it all week. If you are a multicooker user, you can shave the cooking time down to under an hour.

1 onion, halved through the equator

1 whole chicken (3½ to 4 pounds)

2 carrots, scrubbed (unpeeled) and cut into thirds

2 celery stalks, cut into thirds

1 whole head of garlic, cut in half across the equator

1 bay leaf

10 fresh thyme sprigs

½ teaspoon whole black peppercorns

Heat a large pot over medium heat. Place the onion cut side down in the dry, hot pan. Cook for about 5 minutes, or until deep golden brown.

Add the chicken, carrots, celery, garlic, bay leaf, thyme, peppercorns, and 3½ quarts water to the pot. Bring to a simmer over medium-high heat. Skim the top of the broth, discarding any impurities that rise to the surface. Adjust the heat to maintain a gentle simmer and cook the broth for 1 hour, uncovered, skimming as needed. Transfer the chicken to a plate.

Use tongs to remove as much meat as possible from the chicken (be careful, the chicken will be hot!) and set aside. Return the skin, bones, and carcass to the pot and continue to simmer the broth for an additional hour. When it's cool enough to handle, shred the reserved chicken meat into bite-size pieces and refrigerate for up to 5 days or freeze or for up to 1 month. (If freezing, be sure to remove as much air as possible from the container to prevent freezer burn.)

Remove the pot from the heat and strain the broth into pint or quart containers. Discard the bones and vegetables. Allow the broth to cool, then refrigerate for up to 4 days or freeze for up to 3 months.

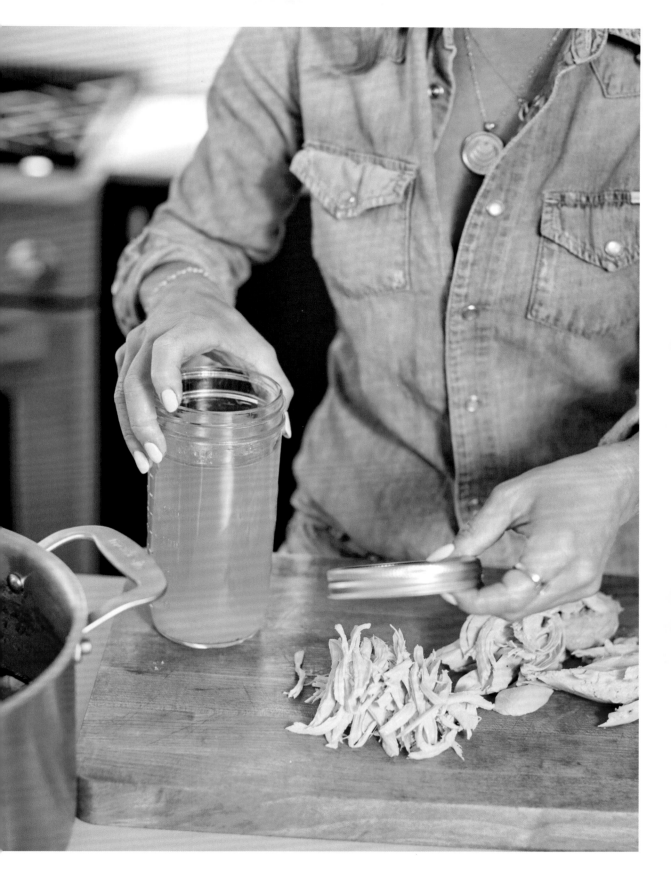

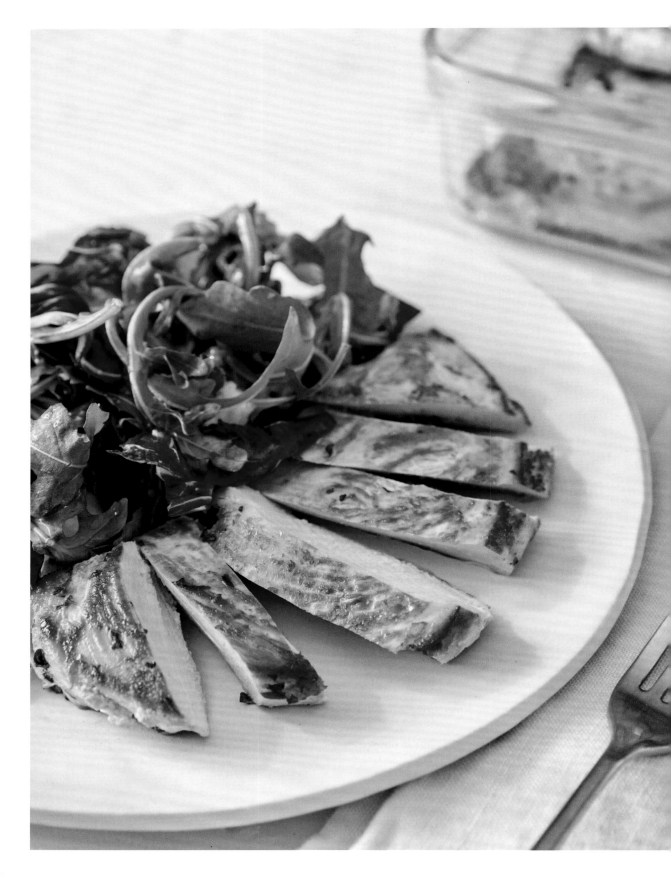

LEMON *and* OREGANO POUNDED CHICKEN

SERVES 4

This marinated, thinly pounded chicken can work in many different ways: as a topper for a salad, in a sandwich, or in a lettuce wrap. I especially love how quickly it cooks. When it's done, store it with its cooking juices and, if it looks like it might be too dry, pour in some extra chicken broth to keep it nice and moist. The chicken does need to marinate for at least four hours, so plan accordingly.

2 tablespoons olive oil

2 teaspoons grated lemon zest, from 2 lemons

1 tablespoon lemon juice, from ½ lemon

2 teaspoons chopped fresh oregano

1¼ teaspoons kosher salt

4 boneless, skinless chicken breasts (about 6 ounces each)

Combine 1 tablespoon of the olive oil, the lemon zest, lemon juice, oregano, and salt in a large resealable plastic bag. Massage the bag to combine the ingredients. Add the chicken breasts, seal the bag, and massage the marinade evenly into the chicken. Press the air out of the bag and reseal. Pound the chicken breasts to flatten them to ½ to ¾ inch thick. Marinate in the refrigerator for at least 4 hours and up to 10 hours.

Remove the chicken from the refrigerator about 15 minutes before cooking.

Heat a skillet large enough to hold the chicken in one layer over medium-high heat. Add the remaining tablespoon of olive oil and swirl to coat the bottom. Add the chicken to the pan, smooth side down, and place something heavy on top to press the breasts onto the hot surface. (A brick wrapped in aluminum foil or a small cast-iron skillet with a piece of foil between it and the chicken works well here.)

Cook the chicken for 5 minutes, or until deep golden brown on the first side. Remove the weight and flip the chicken. Continue to cook for about 5 minutes, or until the breasts are firm to the touch and an instant-read thermometer inserted in the thickest part reads 160°F. Transfer to a storage container. Add ⅓ cup water to the pan to deglaze and pour the juices over the chicken. Refrigerate for up to 5 days or freeze for a month.

OLIVE OIL–POACHED SALMON

SERVES 4

Poaching salmon in oil keeps it so silky and moist, and if you store leftovers in the poaching oil, they won't dry out in the refrigerator. This is not the time to break out that very special bottle of evoo; a supermarket brand will do fine.

4 skinless center-cut salmon fillets (about 5 ounces each)

1 teaspoon whole fennel seeds

3 cups olive oil

3 garlic cloves, smashed and peeled

3 fresh rosemary sprigs

1 bay leaf

1 teaspoon kosher salt

Lemon wedges, for serving

Remove the salmon from the refrigerator 40 minutes before cooking.

Heat a medium straight-sided skillet just large enough to fit all 4 fillets in a single layer. Add the fennel seeds and toast over medium heat for 2 minutes, or until fragrant. Add the oil, garlic, rosemary, and bay leaf. Reduce the heat to medium-low and steep the aromatics in the oil for 10 minutes.

Reduce the heat to low. Place a deep-fry thermometer on the side of the pan and let the temperature of the oil come down to 175°F.

Using paper towels, dry the salmon well and season on all sides with the salt. Slide the salmon into the warm oil. The salmon should be completely covered by the oil. Poach for 15 to 20 minutes, until opaque all the way through and firm to the touch. The salmon is now ready to serve or store. To serve, use a wide metal spatula to lift the fillets out of the oil and transfer to a paper-towel-lined tray to drain. Serve the freshly cooked salmon warm with lemon wedges, or allow the fish and the oil it was cooked in to cool and transfer to a storage container. The oil-covered salmon will keep for 3 or 4 days in the refrigerator and can be served cold at room temperature or gently reheated.

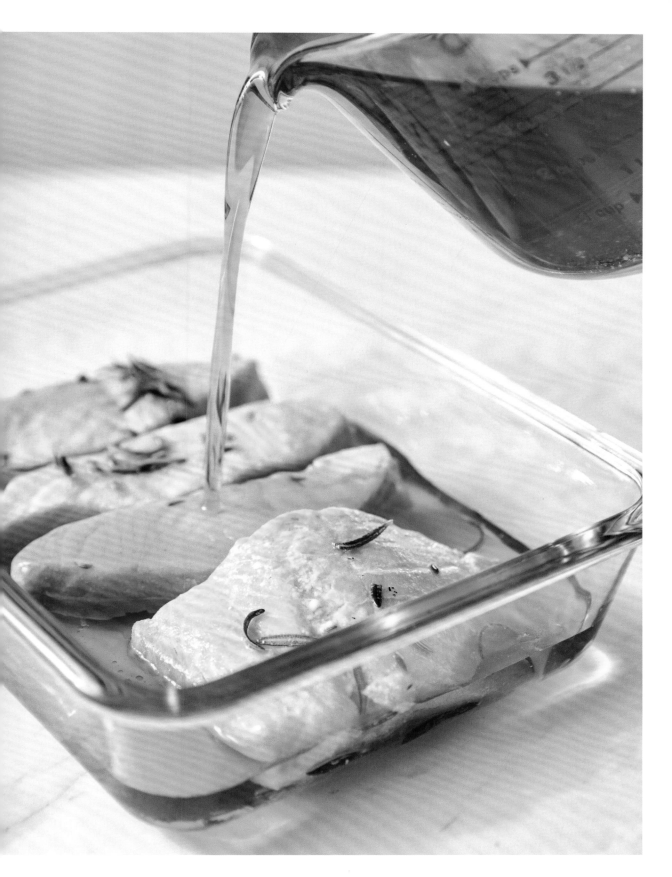

CHAPTER 9

Breakfast

Big breakfasts aren't really a thing in Italy the way they are in other countries, and as a kid I usually just grabbed a piece of bread before heading out the door. I still prefer to keep breakfast on the lighter side—eating too much that early in the day just makes me start dragging by midmorning—but now I like to have a little protein and fiber along with my carbs.

Smoothies or a chia pudding or yogurt parfait are my go-tos for the days I want something light and fast, and they make good anytime snacks too. On the weekends, though, I do give in to my weakness for starchier things like pancakes and warm cereals. I find that a reasonable amount of carbs for breakfast—by which I mean three or four pancakes, not a towering stack drenched in syrup—is really comforting and keeps me satisfied longer. But I make an effort to use added sweeteners sparingly in all of these recipes, so I'm not starting my day on a sugar high. However you like to fuel yourself for the day ahead, you will find a delicious option here.

ALMOND MILK

MAKES 3 CUPS

It may sound intimidating to make almond milk from scratch, but nothing could be easier; all you need is a blender and a few hours of hands-off soaking time. It's actually empowering to make something this basic yourself, and if you will be making it often, invest in a nut-milk bag, which I think works better than cheesecloth. In a pinch you can also use an old (clean) pillowcase!

1 cup raw almonds

Pinch of kosher salt (optional)

Place the raw almonds in a bowl with enough water to cover by 2 inches. Soak the almonds at room temperature for 4 hours or overnight in the refrigerator.

Drain the almonds and rinse them well under cold water. Add the soaked almonds and 3 cups water to a blender along with the salt, if using. Puree on high for 2 minutes, or until smooth and creamy. Strain the mixture through a nut-milk bag or a fine-mesh strainer lined with three layers of cheesecloth, pressing on the solids to extract as much liquid as possible. Store the almond milk in an airtight container in the refrigerator for up to 3 days.

VEGGIE-BERRY BREAKFAST SMOOTHIE

This is especially rich and creamy made with your own fresh almond milk. If using store-bought, be sure your brand contains only almonds, water, and salt; many commercial brands contain flavorings, sweeteners, and thickeners like carrageenan. I make this on the weekend when I want a little sustenance before going for a hike or to a yoga class but don't want to feel too full. That little bit of coconut oil really gives it staying power. (See photograph on page 106.)

1 cup frozen blueberries

1 celery stalk, chopped

½ cup peeled and chopped English cucumber

2 tablespoons peeled and chopped fresh ginger

1 cup baby arugula

½ avocado

1 tablespoon coconut oil

1 cup unsweetened almond milk, homemade (page 104) or store-bought

½ cup ice

Pinch of kosher salt

Combine the blueberries, celery, cucumber, ginger, arugula, avocado, coconut oil, almond milk, ½ cup water, the ice, and salt in a blender. Blend on high speed until completely smooth, about 1½ minutes. Divide between two glasses and serve.

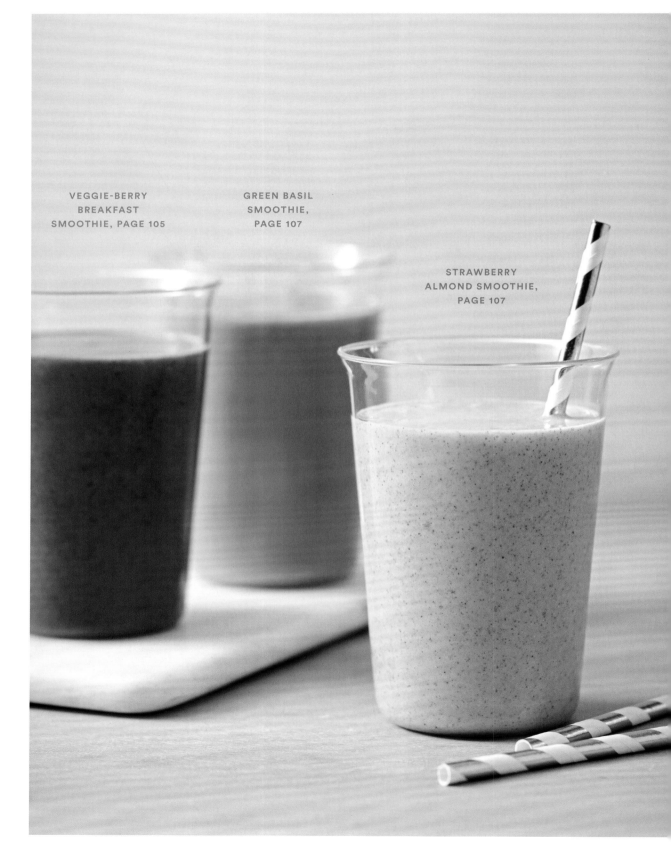

VEGGIE-BERRY
BREAKFAST
SMOOTHIE, PAGE 105

GREEN BASIL
SMOOTHIE,
PAGE 107

STRAWBERRY
ALMOND SMOOTHIE,
PAGE 107

GREEN BASIL SMOOTHIE

MAKES TWO 14-OUNCE SMOOTHIES

Italians don't really go for smoothies the way we do here, but if they did, I think this one would be their top pick. It's just sweet enough and full of green goodness with a hint of basil.

2 cups (packed) baby spinach

1 cup peeled and chopped English cucumber

½ avocado

1 Fuji apple, cored and diced

¼ cup whole raw almonds

¼ cup (packed) fresh basil leaves

1 tablespoon fresh lemon juice, from ½ lemon

1 cup ice cubes

Pinch of kosher salt

Combine the spinach, cucumber, avocado, apple, almonds, basil, lemon juice, 1 cup water, the ice, and the salt in a blender. Blend on high speed for 1½ minutes, or until completely smooth. Divide between two tall glasses and serve.

STRAWBERRY ALMOND SMOOTHIE

MAKES TWO 12-OUNCE SMOOTHIES

This indulgent smoothie really sticks to your ribs thanks to the almond butter. You can soak the chia seeds the night before or just omit them if you're in a hurry, but they do contribute a silky texture and some key fatty acids.

1½ teaspoons chia seeds

¾ cup unsweetened coconut water or unsweetened coconut milk beverage

1 cup frozen strawberries

2 tablespoons unsweetened raw almond butter

1 ripe banana

½ cup ice

Pinch of kosher salt

Stir the chia seeds and coconut water together in a small bowl and let sit for 20 minutes. Pour the soaked seeds and coconut water into a blender, then add the strawberries, almond butter, banana, ice, and salt and puree on high for 1 minute, or until smooth.

COFFEE *and* SPINACH SMOOTHIE

When I serve this smoothie for brunch, it wows people every time. You barely taste the spinach, but you get a little jolt from the coffee. The cocoa nibs are my favorite part! I like to mix up all the ingredients except the ice the night before, so in the morning all I need to do is whiz it with ice just before serving.

1 ripe banana

1 cup unsweetened almond milk, homemade (page 104), or store-bought

2 cups baby spinach

2 cups ice

½ teaspoon pure vanilla extract

Pinch of kosher salt

½ ripe avocado

1 tablespoon finely ground espresso or coffee

1 tablespoon cocoa nibs

Combine the banana, almond milk, spinach, ice, vanilla, and salt in a blender. Puree on high speed for 1 minute, or until almost smooth. Add the avocado and puree for another 30 seconds, or until smooth. Add the coffee and cocoa nibs and pulse to combine. Divide between two glasses and serve.

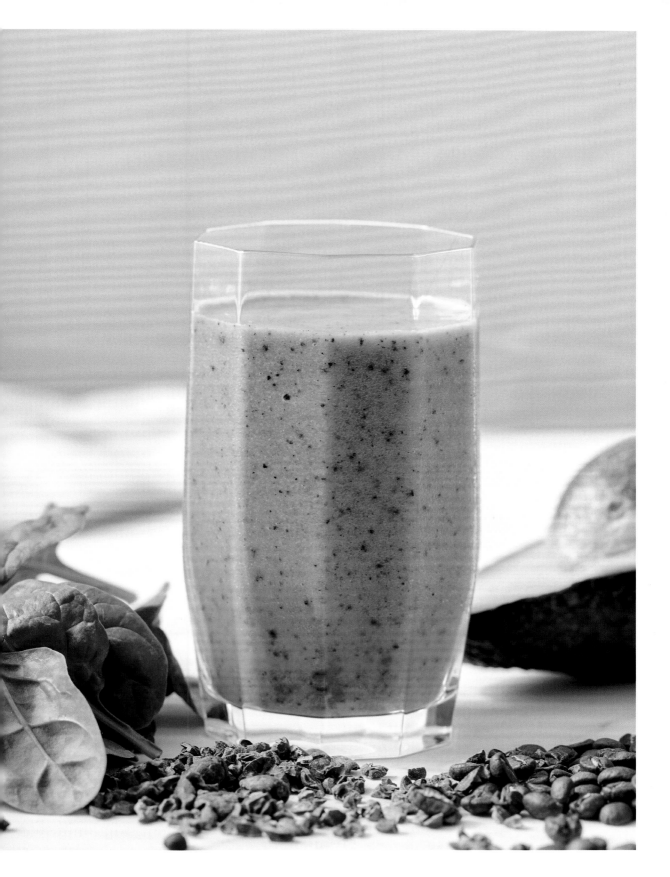

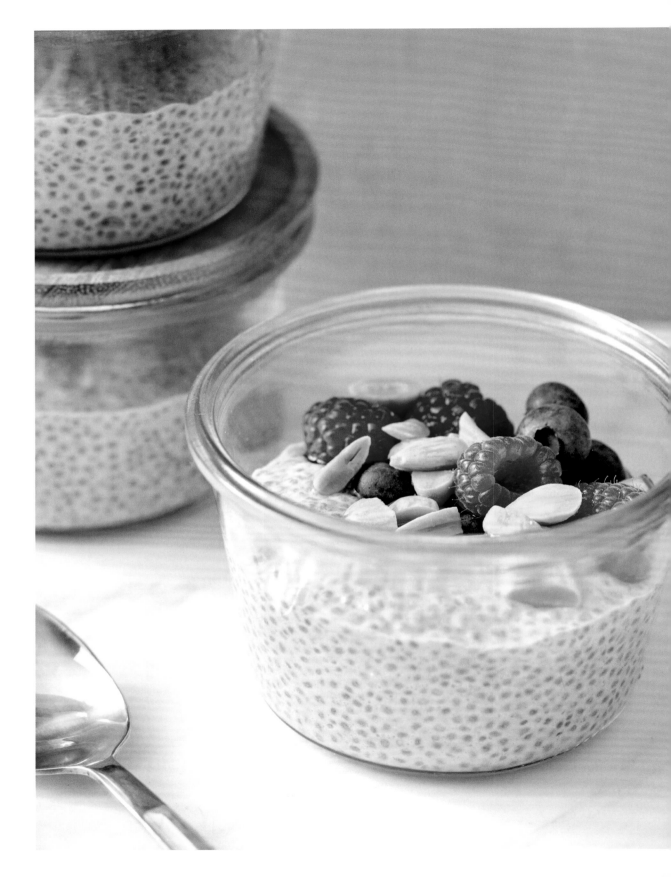

BREAKFAST CHIA SEED PUDDING

SERVES 6

The best part about chia pudding is that you *have* to make it the night before, so in the morning you wake up to a beautiful, ready-to-eat treat. At Pronto, my quick-service restaurant in Las Vegas, these sell out every day; we just can't make enough! I love the richness you get from a sprinkle of Marcona almonds—the kind cooked in olive oil and salt—but even topped with plain toasted almonds, or none at all, this is a lovely breakfast.

2 cups unsweetened almond milk, homemade (page 104), or store-bought

½ cup plus 2 tablespoons chia seeds

1 teaspoon pure vanilla extract

½ teaspoon ground cinnamon

2 tablespoons pure maple syrup

Pinch of kosher salt

¾ cup blueberries

⅓ cup chopped Marcona almonds or toasted almonds

Extra-virgin olive oil, for drizzling (optional)

In a medium bowl, whisk together the almond milk, chia seeds, vanilla, cinnamon, maple syrup, and salt. Allow to sit for 5 minutes at room temperature. Whisk again to fully combine. Cover and refrigerate overnight.

To serve, divide the chia pudding among six bowls. Top with the blueberries and almonds and drizzle each serving with ½ teaspoon olive oil, if desired.

COCONUT YOGURT PARFAIT

MAKES 1 PARFAIT

Another top seller at Pronto, which offers healthier, quality foods in a fast-service environment, this parfait is so much better than a plain cup of (sugary) flavored yogurt. It works equally well as a breakfast or a simple dessert. Use whichever berries are in season, look best, or are on sale! If you can find a local honey to drizzle on top, so much the better.

½ cup plain coconut yogurt or 2% plain Greek yogurt

⅓ cup Maple and Olive Oil Quinoa Granola (page 114) or your favorite store-bought granola

2 pitted dates, chopped (optional)

1 tablespoon chopped tart dried cherries

¼ cup mixed fresh berries, such as blueberries and raspberries

Drizzle of honey (optional)

In a parfait glass or small bowl, layer half the yogurt, half the granola, and all the chopped dates, if using, and cherries. Top with the remaining yogurt and granola and the berries. Drizzle with some honey, if desired, and serve.

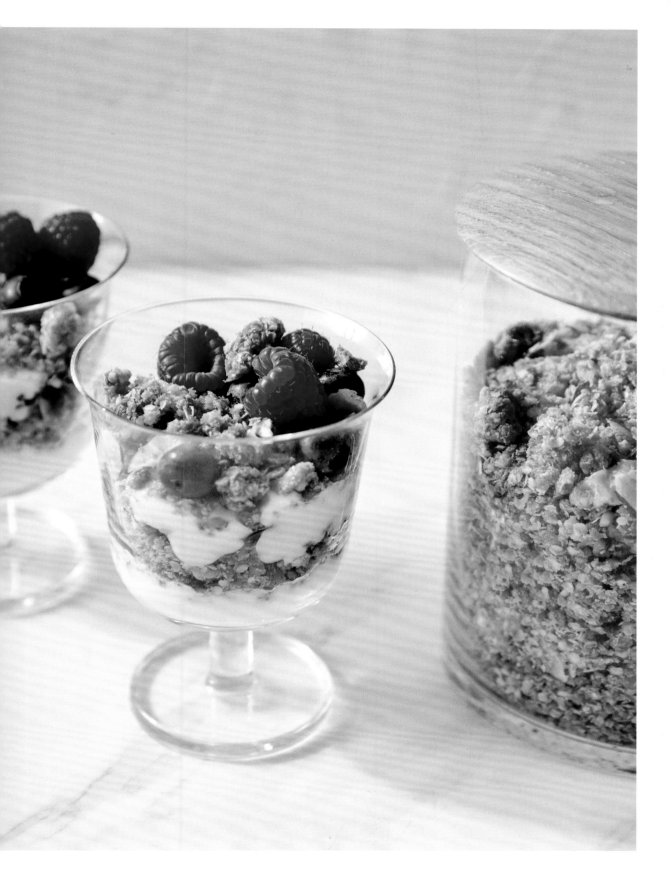

MAPLE *and* OLIVE OIL QUINOA GRANOLA

MAKES 7 CUPS

It's important to have sensible snack items around when you are trying to eat cleaner, so I always make this granola in big batches. I add it to my nut mix or eat it out of hand, sprinkle it on yogurt for a fast snack or light meal, or toss some into a salad for a little added sweetness and crunch. (See photograph on page 113.)

5 cups quinoa flakes
(see Note)

1 cup pure maple syrup

¾ cup olive oil

2 teaspoons pure vanilla
extract

2 teaspoons kosher salt

1 cup chopped walnuts

1 cup sliced almonds

Preheat the oven to 350°F. Line a rimmed baking sheet with parchment paper and set aside.

In a large bowl, mix together the quinoa flakes, maple syrup, olive oil, vanilla, salt, and walnuts. Toss well to coat evenly. Spread the mixture on the prepared baking sheet and bake for 30 minutes, stirring once after 15 minutes. Remove the pan from the oven and stir in the almonds. Bake for an additional 25 to 30 minutes, stirring once again halfway through to brown evenly. Remove from the oven and let the granola cool completely on the baking sheet. Store in an airtight container for up to 3 weeks.

NOTE ────────

Quinoa flakes are made from quinoa grains that have been rolled and flattened—just like rolled oats. Check for them near the hot cereals and make sure what you are buying is 100 percent quinoa, not a breakfast cereal.

OLIVE OIL–SCRAMBLED EGGS WITH ARUGULA *and* FENNEL SALAD

SERVES 2

Starting the day with a big plate of greens and eggs just makes me smile and gives me all the fuel I need to go right through lunch. This would more likely be a light supper in Italy, and when I'm on my own, I sometimes make this in the evening to enjoy with a spritzer or a glass of Prosecco on ice.

FOR THE SALAD

2 cups baby arugula

½ fennel bulb, stalks removed, thinly sliced

1 teaspoon fresh lemon juice

1½ teaspoons extra-virgin olive oil

¼ teaspoon kosher salt

FOR THE EGGS

4 large eggs

½ teaspoon kosher salt

2 tablespoons olive oil

Freshly ground black pepper (optional)

In a medium bowl, combine the arugula, fennel, lemon juice, extra-virgin olive oil, and salt. Toss gently to combine. Divide between two plates.

Crack the eggs into a medium bowl. Add the salt and whisk until smooth and completely combined. Heat a medium nonstick skillet over medium-low heat. Add the oil and heat for another minute. Add the egg mixture to the hot oil. Using a rubber spatula, stir the eggs constantly, shaking the pan occasionally to help keep the eggs moving. When the eggs look almost cooked but are still creamy and slightly wet, remove the pan from the heat. Continue to stir the eggs off the heat for about 3 minutes, or until done to your liking. Take your time here and be patient. Divide the eggs between the two plates, top with a few grinds of pepper if you like, and serve.

ASPARAGUS SCRAMBLE

SERVES 2

This reminds me of the kind of elegant brunch dish you would get at a country club, maybe with a slice of smoked salmon draped over the top—except you're making it in the comfort of your own kitchen (no dress code required). If you are an asparagus lover, this will be right up your alley, but don't limit yourself; you can really use any leftover vegetable you have. The flecks of green from the asparagus and chives make it an especially pretty Sunday breakfast.

2 tablespoons olive oil

½ bunch of asparagus, ends trimmed, cut into ¼-inch pieces

½ teaspoon kosher salt

4 large eggs

1½ tablespoons chopped chives

Freshly ground black pepper (optional)

Heat a medium nonstick skillet over medium heat. Add the olive oil and heat for an additional minute. Add the asparagus and ¼ teaspoon of the salt. Cook, stirring often with a rubber spatula, until the asparagus is tender, about 4 minutes.

While the asparagus cooks, in a medium bowl, whisk together the eggs, the remaining ¼ teaspoon salt, and 1 tablespoon of the chives.

When the asparagus is tender, reduce the heat to low. Add the egg mixture to the pan and stir in long, slow strokes, using the rubber spatula to scrape the set eggs up from the bottom of the pan and allow the loose egg to cook. When the mixture is almost set but still slightly wet, about 1 minute, turn off the heat. Continue to stir off the heat until the mixture is creamy and just set, about 3 minutes. Serve sprinkled with the remaining ½ tablespoon chives and a bit of black pepper, if desired.

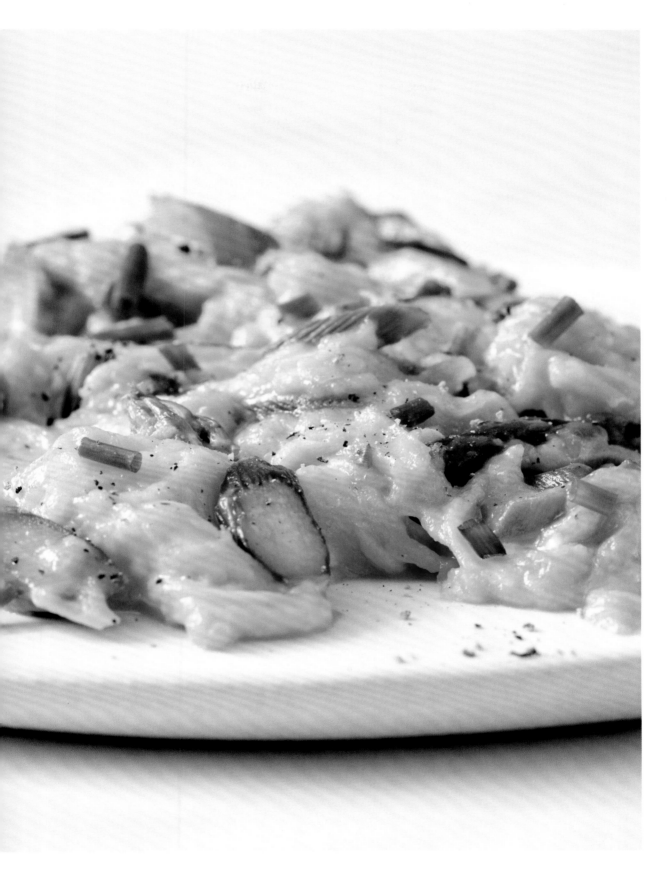

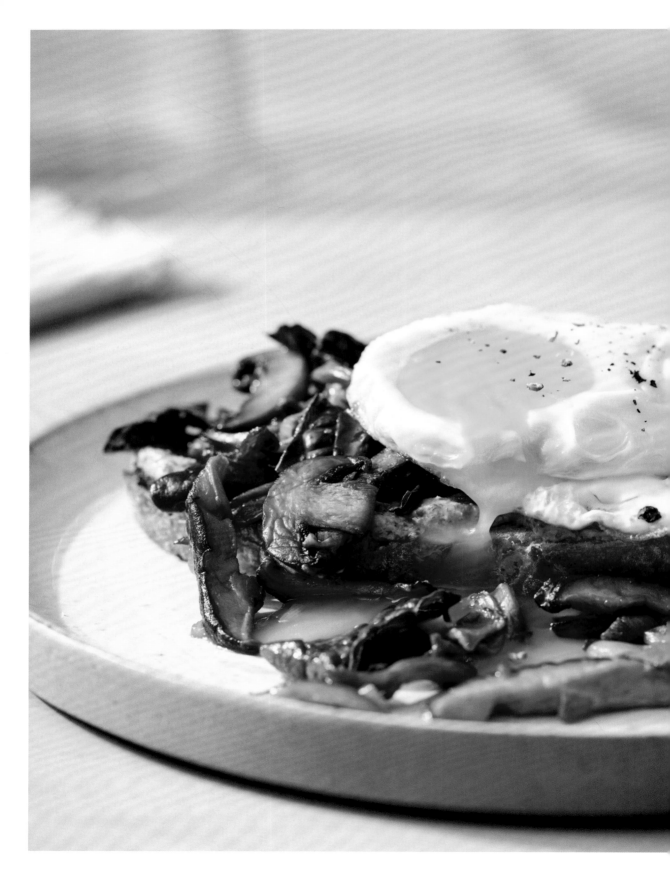

MUSHROOM TOAST

SERVES 4

This is no two-biter, like a crostini; it's a sophisticated, sexy dish that's perfect for brunch, lunch, or even a lighter dinner. Kale, mushrooms, and earthy Marsala wine make it super savory and meaty. The eggs, while not mandatory, bind all the elements together into a creamy, delicious mouthful.

5 tablespoons olive oil

1 pound assorted mushrooms, such as cremini, shiitake, or oyster

1½ teaspoons kosher salt

1 shallot, chopped

1 small bunch of Tuscan kale, tough stems discarded, chopped

3 tablespoons dry Marsala, sherry, or red wine

1½ tablespoons unsalted butter, preferably European-style

4 (1-inch-thick) slices of rustic bread, gluten-free if desired, toasted

¼ cup whole-grain mustard

4 large eggs

Heat a large nonstick skillet over medium-high heat. Add 3 tablespoons of the olive oil. Add the mushrooms to the hot oil, season with ¾ teaspoon of the salt, and cook, stirring occasionally, for 10 minutes, or until deep golden brown. Add the shallot and cook for an additional 3 minutes, stirring constantly. Add the kale and ¼ teaspoon of the salt and cook for another 2 minutes, or until the kale is wilted. Remove from the heat and add the Marsala, using a wooden spoon to scrape up the brown bits from the bottom of the pan. Add the butter and stir until it is incorporated into the sauce.

Spread each slice of toast with a tablespoon of the mustard. Divide the mushroom mixture evenly among the toasts.

Wipe out the pan with a paper towel and return it to the stovetop over medium heat. Add the remaining 2 tablespoons olive oil and, when hot, carefully break the eggs into the pan. Season with the remaining ½ teaspoon salt. Cook over medium heat until the whites are set and browned around the edges but the yolks are still runny, 3 to 4 minutes, spooning some of the hot oil over the whites if they need help setting. Top each toast with an egg and serve.

WARM QUINOA "OATMEAL"

SERVES 2

For the longest time my everyday breakfast was cooked brown rice with a little olive oil and salt because regular oatmeal doesn't always agree with me. Now I've switched to this homey, comforting breakfast, which has a little more sweetness and flavor. I find a pinch of spice gives it a warm, cozy taste and aroma.

1 cup cooked quinoa (page 92)

⅔ cup unsweetened almond milk, homemade (page 104), or store-bought

⅔ cup mixed fruit, such as berries or mango, or unsweetened flaked coconut, or a combination

2 tablespoons sliced almonds

2 teaspoons extra-virgin olive oil or coconut oil

4 teaspoons pure maple syrup

Pinch of flake salt (optional)

Ground cinnamon, ginger, nutmeg, or cardamom (optional)

Add the quinoa and almond milk to a small saucepan. Place over medium heat and bring to a low simmer. Cook for 2 to 3 minutes, just to heat through. Spoon the mixture into two bowls and top with the fruits, nuts, olive oil, and maple syrup. Sprinkle with flake salt and the ground spice, if desired. Serve warm.

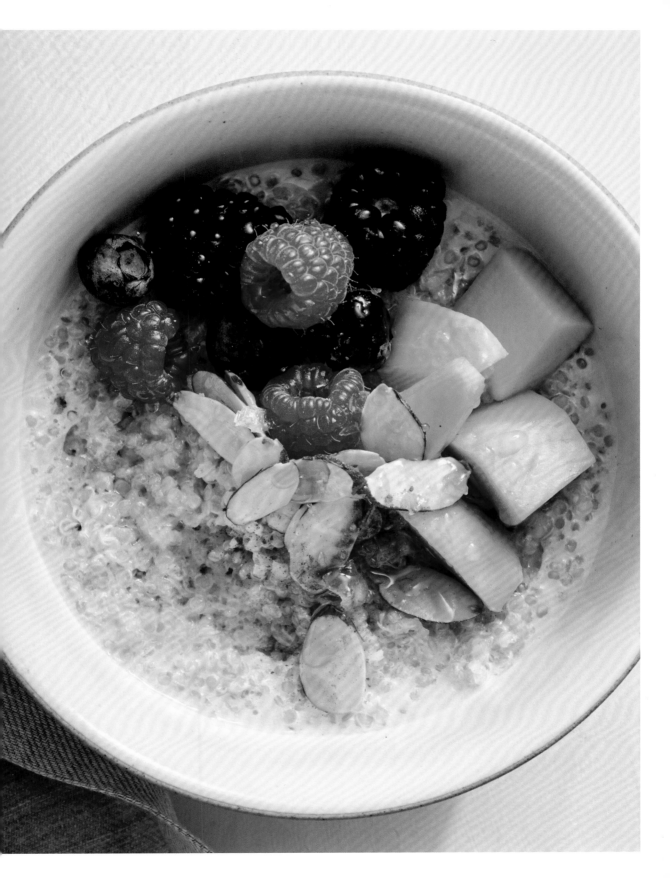

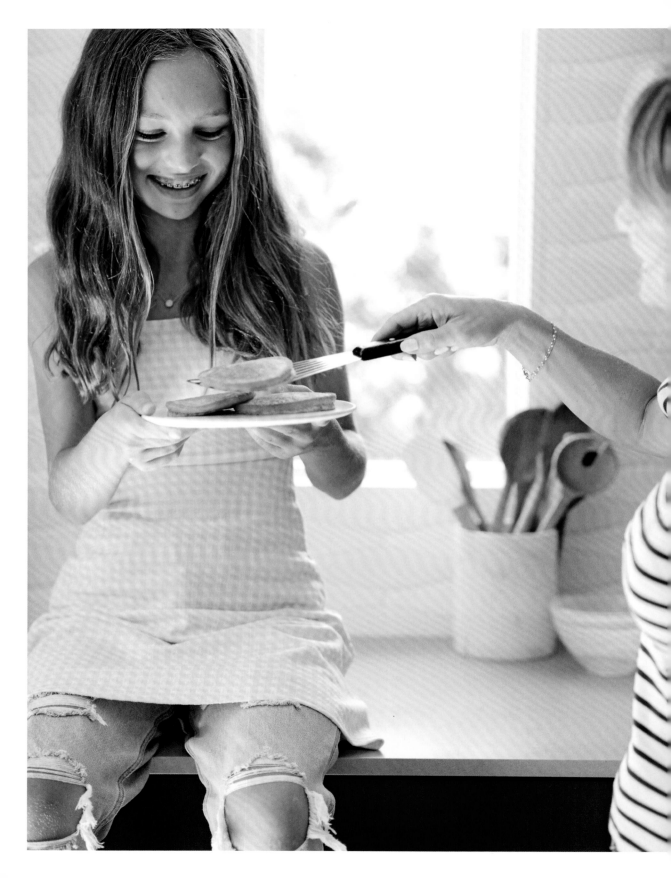

QUINOA PANCAKES

SERVES 4 TO 5

Jade would eat pancakes every day if I let her, so I've started making different kinds, just to mix it up. These are made with white rice flour (or oat flour) instead of wheat flour, so they're gluten-free; they're extra good topped with Mixed Berries with Spiced Maple Syrup (page 257). On the weekends, I've even been known to throw a few chocolate chips into the batter for her. Leftover pancakes (if there are any!) freeze well and can be reheated in the toaster for fast weekday breakfasts.

1 cup rice flour or gluten-free oat flour

1 teaspoon baking powder

½ teaspoon baking soda

¼ teaspoon kosher salt

⅔ cup coconut yogurt, such as COYO

2 large eggs, at room temperature

1 teaspoon pure vanilla extract

1 tablespoon pure maple syrup, plus more for serving

1 cup cooked quinoa, cooled (page 92)

Coconut oil or grapeseed oil, for the pan

Unsalted butter, for serving

In a large bowl, whisk together the flour, baking powder, baking soda, and salt. In a separate bowl, whisk together the coconut yogurt, eggs, vanilla, maple syrup, and ⅓ cup water. Add the wet ingredients to the bowl with the dry and whisk until only a few lumps remain. Fold in the quinoa.

Preheat the oven to 200°F. Heat a large skillet or griddle over medium heat. Brush with a bit of oil, then ladle the batter onto the griddle, using ¼ cup per pancake. Cook for 2 to 3 minutes on the first side, or until little bubbles start to form on the surface. Flip the pancakes and cook for another minute, until lightly browned. Transfer to a plate and place in the oven to keep warm while you make the remaining pancakes.

Serve warm with butter and more maple syrup.

BUCKWHEAT CARDAMOM PANCAKES

SERVES 4

If you are looking for a naturally gluten-free alternative to your usual pancake mix, give these a spin. I like to serve them as part of a brunch buffet. They have a deep, rich color, like blini, with a great nutty flavor and lots of warm spices that make them smell amazing. Cook up a double batch and freeze the extras for quick weekday breakfasts.

½ cup buckwheat flour

½ cup rice flour

½ teaspoon baking powder

½ teaspoon baking soda

¼ teaspoon kosher salt

1 teaspoon ground cardamom

½ teaspoon ground cinnamon

⅔ cup coconut yogurt, such as COYO

2 large eggs, at room temperature

1 teaspoon pure vanilla extract

Coconut oil or grapeseed oil, for the pan

Pure maple syrup and berries, for serving

In a medium bowl, whisk together the buckwheat flour, rice flour, baking powder, baking soda, salt, cardamom, and cinnamon. Make a well in the center and add the yogurt, ⅓ cup water, the eggs, and vanilla. Starting in the center, use a whisk to break up the eggs, then whisk the dry ingredients into the wet until the batter is smooth and only a few lumps remain.

Heat a large skillet or griddle over medium heat. Brush the surface of the pan with oil. Working in batches, spoon the batter onto the pan, using a scant ¼ cup for each pancake. Cook for 1 minute on the first side, or until bubbles start to form on the top. Flip the pancakes and cook for an additional minute to cook through. Transfer to a plate and cover to keep warm while you cook the remaining pancakes. Serve warm with maple syrup and berries.

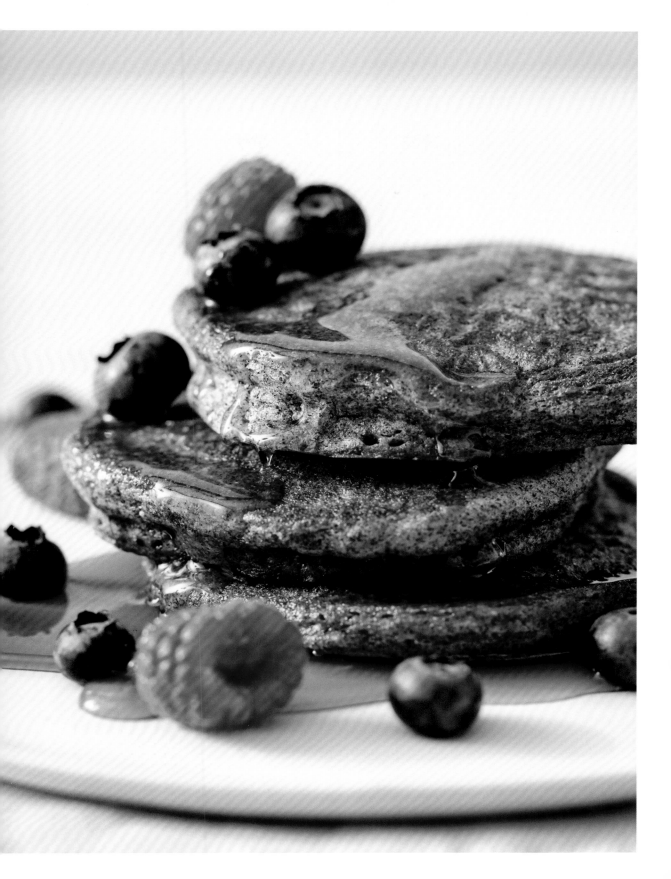

CHAPTER 10

Lean and Clean

Two or three times each year I like to eat especially clean for a few days to give my digestion a chance to recover from overindulgence or to put myself back on a better path (see pages 57–63 for more about my three-day reboot meal plan). That's when the recipes in this chapter, an all-day assortment of snacks, soups, and one-dish meals, are in especially heavy rotation.

You won't find anything from the Proceed with Caution list (page 23) in these recipes, just lots and lots of nutrient-rich veggies, a reasonable amount of lean proteins, and only enough whole grains to keep your energy level high and your belly full. But don't dismiss these recipes as too austere for every day; I find many of them just right for those nights when all I want to do is curl up in front of the TV with a bowl of something savory and binge my favorite shows. Give these recipes a try, and I bet you'll add them to your weekly roster too.

CELERY WATER

SERVES 2

You don't need a fancy juicer to make this pureed celery drink, which has become popular for its detoxifying and anti-inflammatory properties. I find it refreshing and not too filling. A high-speed blender or smoothie maker will break down the stalks into a perfectly smooth liquid. If your blender isn't quite that powerful, blend it a bit longer and then strain out any remaining fibrous bits.

2 celery stalks, roughly chopped

1 tablespoon fresh lemon juice, from ½ lemon

Pinch of kosher salt

Combine the celery, lemon juice, and salt in a blender. Add 1 cup cold water and blend on high speed for 1 minute, or until completely pureed and smooth. Serve immediately.

GREEN REFRESHER

MAKES TWO 12-OUNCE SMOOTHIES

Try this after your next workout as a rehydrating replenisher that leans more savory than sweet. I also like it as a between-meal snack or even in place of a salad! You can make it ahead of time, pureeing everything but the ice in a blender, then whizzing the puree with ice just before serving. Alternatively, divide everything but the water and ice between two zip-top freezer bags—avocado and all—and freeze. Then just pop the contents of a bag into the blender along with 1 cup water. Easy!

2 small romaine hearts, chopped

½ fennel bulb, trimmed and chopped

½ avocado

1 celery stalk, chopped

1 cup ice

Pinch of kosher salt

In a blender, combine the romaine, fennel, avocado, celery, ice, and salt with 1 cup water. Blend on high speed until completely smooth, about 1½ minutes. Pour into two tall glasses and serve.

WALNUT GARLIC DIP

If you can make hummus, you can make this nutty, lemony dip. Jade likes it with some colorful cut-up vegetables as an after-school snack; I think the walnuts make it especially tasty with endive spears for scooping. If it's not a reboot day, top this with a couple tablespoons of crumbled feta. (See photograph on page 130.)

1½ cups toasted walnuts (see Note)

1 garlic clove, smashed and peeled

1 teaspoon kosher salt

½ cup cooked white beans (page 90) or canned beans, drained and rinsed

1 teaspoon grated lemon zest

1 tablespoon fresh lemon juice, from ½ lemon

¼ cup extra-virgin olive oil, plus more to drizzle

2 tablespoons chopped fresh mint

Crudités, for serving

In the bowl of a food processor, combine the walnuts, garlic, and salt. Pulse until finely chopped. Add the white beans, lemon zest, lemon juice, olive oil, and ¼ cup water and puree until smooth. Add the mint and pulse to combine.

Serve drizzled with a bit of extra-virgin olive oil and lots of veggies for dipping.

NOTE ———————

To toast the walnuts, spread them evenly on a rimmed baking sheet and bake in a 400°F oven for 8 minutes. Transfer to a plate to cool to prevent them from getting too dark.

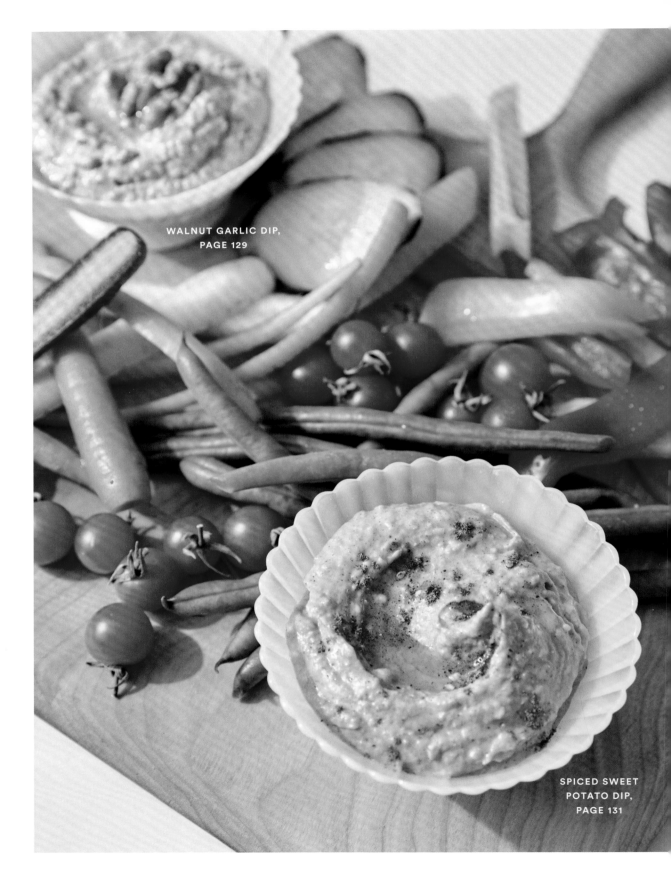

WALNUT GARLIC DIP,
PAGE 129

SPICED SWEET
POTATO DIP,
PAGE 131

SPICED SWEET POTATO DIP

SERVES 6

A little zippier and a whole lot prettier than regular hummus, this version is also quite filling. I've seasoned it with za'atar, a Middle Eastern blend of seasonings that includes dried herbs, cumin, and sesame seeds. If you don't have za'atar, you can substitute ¼ teaspoon cumin. Keep it covered until right before you serve it, as the surface dries out if left exposed to the air.

1 sweet potato (about ¾ pound)

⅓ cup olive oil

2 garlic cloves, smashed and peeled

1 cup canned chickpeas, drained

¼ cup almond butter (see Note)

1 tablespoon fresh lemon juice, from ½ lemon

2 teaspoons kosher salt

½ teaspoon za'atar

Extra-virgin olive oil, for drizzling

Crudités, for serving

Preheat the oven to 400°F.

Place the sweet potato on a rimmed baking sheet and pierce it a few times with the tip of a knife. Bake the potato for about 1 hour, until tender all the way through. Allow to cool slightly.

In a small skillet, warm the oil and garlic over low heat for about 10 minutes, until the garlic is lightly browned and soft. Set aside to cool.

Combine the chickpeas, almond butter, lemon juice, salt, and cooled garlic and olive oil in a food processor. Puree until smooth. Scoop the flesh of the sweet potato into the processor and puree again until combined and smooth.

Transfer the hummus to a bowl and sprinkle with the za'atar. Stir in briefly, leaving a little swirl visible. Serve drizzled with olive oil and surrounded by crudités.

NOTE ———————

The brand of almond butter I use is made from lightly toasted nuts, which adds a nice flavor, but any kind will do.

HARD-BOILED EGGS
TWO WAYS

SERVES 4 TO 6

Keeping a few hard-boiled eggs in the fridge is always a smart idea, especially for those days when you'll be out and about but don't have time to pack
a lunch. The problem is that they are not always the most exciting things to
eat. Enter these two boldly flavored condiments, one made with curry and
avocado, the other a Mediterranean-influenced blend of olives accented
with basil and orange zest. Either will transform those handy eggs into
something super tasty. At home, you can make a lunch of it by quartering
the eggs and serving them over greens and chopped raw veggies dolloped
with either condiment.

8 large eggs

FOR THE AVOCADO MASH

1 ripe avocado

½ teaspoon curry powder

½ teaspoon fresh lemon
    juice

⅓ teaspoon kosher salt

FOR THE OLIVE SPREAD

½ cup mixed pitted olives

2 tablespoons chopped
    fresh basil

½ teaspoon grated orange
    zest

2 teaspoons olive oil

Place the eggs in a small saucepan and cover with water. Bring to a
boil over medium-high heat. Remove from the heat and set aside,
covered, for 10 minutes. Drain the eggs and drop them in a bowl of
ice water.

While the eggs cool, make a topping. For the avocado mash,
combine the avocado, curry powder, lemon juice, and salt in a
medium bowl. Mash with the back of a fork until smooth.

To make the olive spread, combine the olives, basil, orange zest,
and olive oil in a food processor. Pulse just until finely chopped; you
don't want to make a puree.

Carefully peel and halve the eggs. Serve the eggs with one or both of
the condiments.

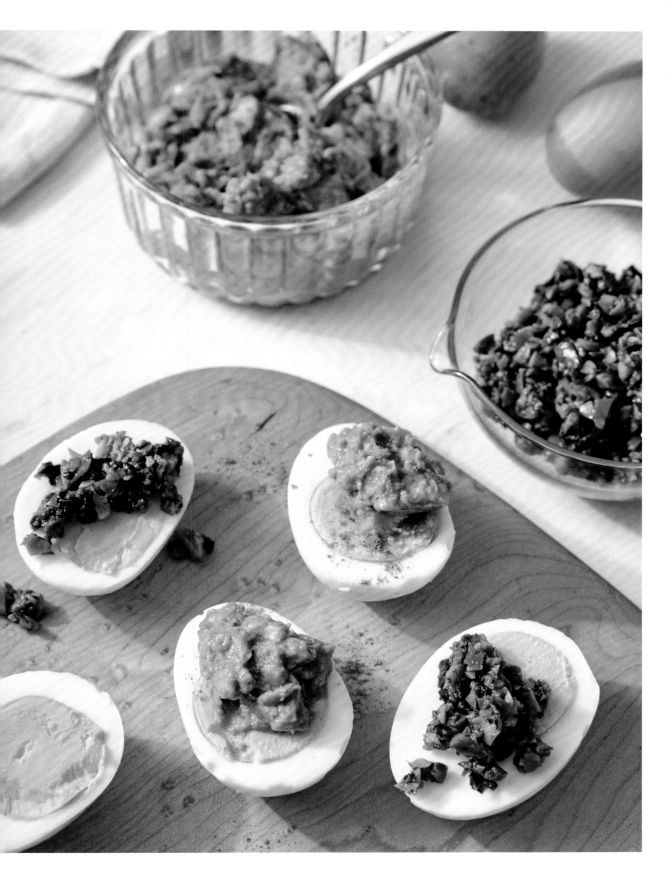

CREAMY CAULIFLOWER SOUP WITH PEPITAS

SERVES 6

This is a vegan version of a cauliflower soup we serve at my restaurant in Las Vegas. The smoky pepita garnish is everything: it gives the silky soup such a nice crunch. Both the bit of pureed sweet potato and the touch of coconut oil added at the end give the soup an unctuous creaminess that makes it feel luxurious. Serve it with a bright, sharp salad, like the Simple Salad of Bitter Greens (page 218), for contrast.

2 tablespoons olive oil

1 shallot, chopped

2 teapoons kosher salt

1 large sweet potato, peeled and cut into 1-inch dice

1 large head of cauliflower, cut into 1-inch florets

1 bay leaf

2 cups vegetable broth, homemade (page 95) or low-sodium store-bought

1 tablespoon coconut oil

FOR THE GARNISH

2 teaspoons virgin coconut oil, warmed slightly, or olive oil

⅓ cup raw pumpkin seeds (pepitas)

½ teaspoon smoked paprika

¼ teaspoon kosher salt

Heat a 4-quart Dutch oven over medium heat. Add the olive oil and swirl to coat the bottom. Add the shallot and cook, stirring often, for 1 minute. Season with 1 teaspoon of the salt. Add the sweet potato and cook for another minute, stirring often. Add the cauliflower, bay leaf, vegetable broth, and 3 cups water and bring to a simmer. Reduce the heat to medium-low to maintain a gentle simmer and cook for about 20 minutes, stirring occasionally, until the vegetables are tender.

Meanwhile, make the garnish: preheat the oven to 400°F. Line a small rimmed baking sheet with parchment paper and line a plate with a paper towel.

In a small bowl, toss together the coconut oil, pumpkin seeds, paprika, and ¼ teaspoon salt. Spread on the prepared pan and toast for 8 minutes, stirring halfway through. Transfer the seeds to the plate to drain.

When all the vegetables are tender, remove the bay leaf and discard. Remove the soup from the heat. Using a stick blender, puree on high for about 2 minutes, until smooth and creamy (or transfer the soup to a blender in batches and puree). Add the coconut oil and remaining teaspoon of salt and puree again to incorporate. Serve topped with the spiced pepitas.

HERBY CHICKEN NOODLE SOUP

SERVES 4

I flat-out love chicken soup and consider it one of the most comforting foods on the planet. This one is superclean and green, and gluten-free thanks to the rice noodles, perfect for a reboot day or anytime you want something extra light and fresh. The herbs are not just for garnish; they contribute lots of flavor, so don't skimp on them! If you've gotten in the habit of making your own Two-Fer Chicken Broth (page 96), you'll already have the shredded, cooked chicken on hand, in which case this steamy bowlful can be on the table in about fifteen minutes.

4 ounces pad Thai rice noodles

2 tablespoons olive oil

1 carrot, chopped fine

1 celery stalk, chopped fine

1 teaspoon kosher salt

5 cups chicken broth, homemade (page 96) or low-sodium store-bought

2 cups cooked shredded chicken

1 cup chopped greens, such as collards, kale, or mustard greens

¼ cup sliced scallions

2 red radishes, thinly sliced (optional)

1 cup (packed) mixed fresh herbs, such as cilantro, Thai basil, and dill

Bring a large pot of water to a boil. Add the noodles, turn off the heat, and let stand until softened but not mushy, about 5 minutes. Drain the noodles, rinse with cool water, and set aside.

Heat a medium Dutch oven over medium-high heat. Add the olive oil, carrot, celery, and salt. Cook, stirring often, for about 3 minutes, or until fragrant. Add the chicken broth and bring to a simmer.

Using tongs, dunk the noodles, a small batch at a time, into the boiling broth just to heat through and then divide them among four bowls. Top with the shredded chicken and greens. Ladle the hot broth over the mixture and top with scallions, radishes (if using), and plenty of mixed herbs.

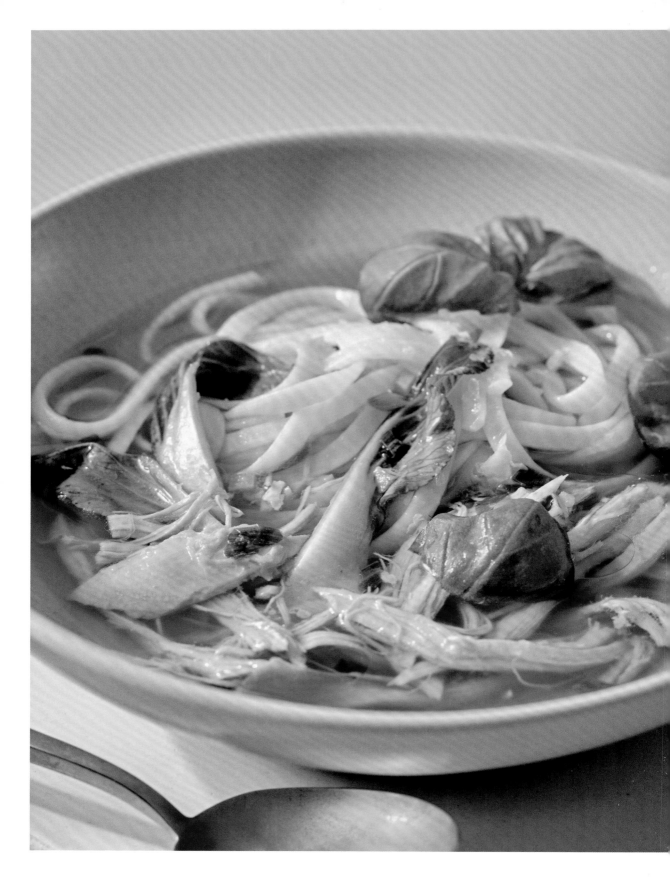

SESAME CHICKEN NOODLE SOUP

SERVES 4

Jade has been really into all kinds of noodles lately, whether it's pho or pad Thai or ramen, but I don't love ordering takeout all the time. This noodle soup brings together many of our favorite notes from pad Thai (the noodles), pho (the herbs), and ramen (the broth). Shred the chicken you cooked to make the chicken broth (page 96) or use leftover rotisserie chicken. If you can find Thai basil (you'll probably have to go to an Asian market), give it a try. Its spicy flavor and unique aroma take this in a whole different direction.

4 ounces rice noodles, such as pad Thai noodles

1 tablespoon dark sesame oil, plus more to drizzle

1 tablespoon olive oil

2 tablespoons peeled and chopped fresh ginger

1 garlic clove, chopped

2 scallions, thinly sliced

1½ cups shredded cooked chicken

1 teaspoon kosher salt

6 cups chicken broth, homemade (page 96) or low-sodium store-bought

1½ tablespoons tamari

2 cups sliced baby bok choy (about 2 heads) or 1 cup small broccoli florets

½ teaspoon flake salt

¼ cup chopped fresh basil or Thai basil

Bring a large pot of water to a boil and season generously with salt. Add the rice noodles and turn off the heat. Let the noodles soften in the hot water just until tender, about 6 minutes, stirring occasionally. Drain the noodles, rinse with cool water, and set aside.

Heat a medium Dutch oven over medium-high heat. Add 1 tablespoon sesame oil and the olive oil and heat for another minute. To the hot pan add the ginger, garlic, and scallions and cook, stirring often with a wooden spoon, until fragrant and soft, about 2 minutes. Add the chicken and salt and stir to coat.

Add the chicken broth to the pot and bring to a boil. Reduce the heat to medium-low and stir in the tamari and bok choy. Simmer for 5 minutes, or until the bok choy is tender and the flavors are combined. Divide the noodles among four bowls and ladle the soup on top. Serve with a drizzle of sesame oil, a sprinkle of flake salt, and some chopped basil.

QUINOA *and* SWEET POTATO STEW-ISH

SERVES 4 TO 6

Soothing and homey, this ragù is a really lovely way to enjoy the flavors and textures of a stew in a meatless meal. The quinoa thickens it up and makes it quite filling. I like the body that the chicken broth lends the stew, but if you prefer a vegan entrée, simply substitute vegetable broth. As long as you have some kind of greens on hand, this is practically a pantry meal.

2 tablespoons olive oil

1 onion, chopped

2 celery stalks, chopped

1 large carrot, chopped

1 fennel bulb, stalks removed, chopped

2 teaspoons kosher salt

1 sweet potato, peeled and cut into ⅓-inch pieces

¾ teaspoon ground cumin

1 bunch of collards, Tuscan kale, or Swiss chard, tough stems discarded, cut into 1-inch pieces

3 cups low-sodium chicken or vegetable broth, homemade (page 96 or 95) or store-bought

1½ cups cooked quinoa (page 92)

Fresh parsley sprigs, for garnish (optional)

Heat a medium Dutch oven over medium-high heat. Add the olive oil and heat for another minute. Add the onion, celery, carrot, fennel, and 1 teaspoon of the salt and cook, stirring often with a wooden spoon, for about 6 minutes, until the vegetables are soft and fragrant.

Add the sweet potato and the cumin to the pot and stir to combine. Cook for 2 minutes to marry the flavors, then add the greens and the remaining teaspoon of salt (see Note). Cook until the greens are wilted, another 2 to 3 minutes. Add the broth and bring to a boil. Reduce the heat to medium-low and simmer for 5 minutes, stirring occasionally. Stir in the cooked quinoa and warm though. Serve hot, topped with the parsley sprigs, if desired.

NOTE ———————

If using store-bought broth, you may not need the full amount of salt. Taste first and then season as needed.

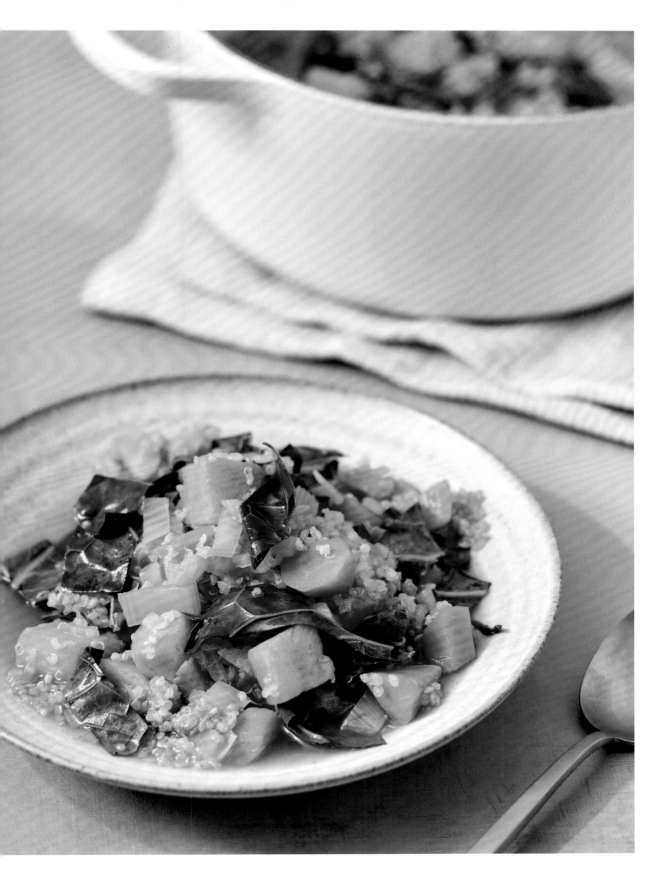

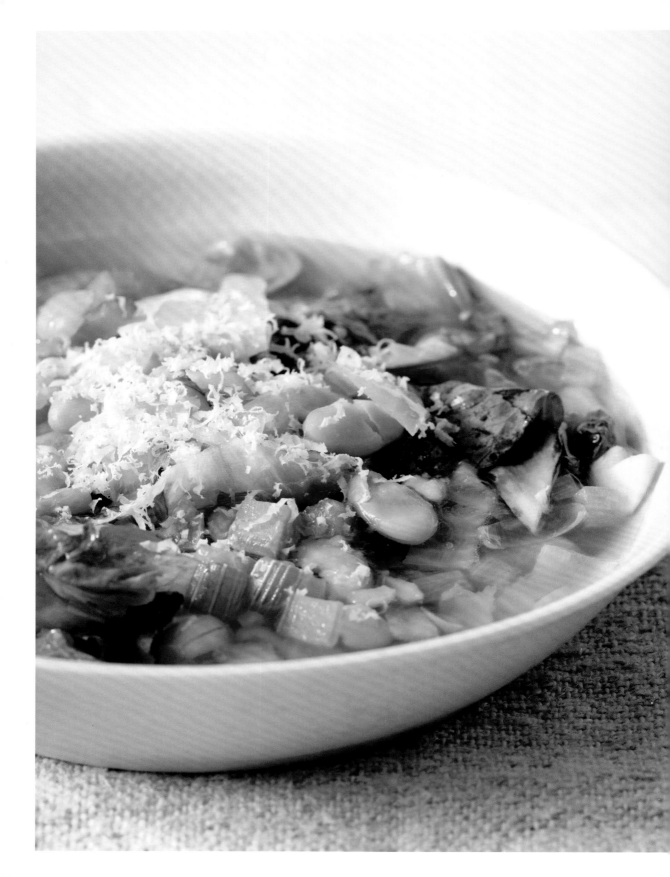

WHITE BEAN
and ESCAROLE SOUP

SERVES 4

We ate this a lot when I was growing up and though I didn't exactly love it
then, it has become something I absolutely crave now. If you have a piece of
Parm rind and are OK with a little dairy, toss it in along with the broth—it will
add depth to the soup. When it's cold outside, there's nothing better.

2 tablespoons olive oil,
   plus more to drizzle

1 onion, chopped

1 celery stalk, chopped

1 carrot, chopped

2 garlic cloves, smashed
   and peeled

1½ teaspoons kosher salt

½ teaspoon crushed red
   pepper flakes (optional)

2½ cups cooked cannellini
   beans (page 90), with
   about ¼ cup cooking
   liquid (see Note)

4 cups chicken broth,
   homemade (page 96)
   or low-sodium
   store-bought

1 head of escarole or
   5 cups baby spinach,
   chopped

Fennel pollen, for garnish
   (optional)

Freshly grated Parmigiano-
   Reggiano, for garnish
   (optional; omit if using
   for a reboot meal)

Heat a medium Dutch oven over medium-high heat. Add
2 tablespoons olive oil, the onion, celery, carrot, and garlic. Season
with the salt and cook, stirring often, for about 4 minutes, until
fragrant and soft. Add the red pepper flakes, if using, and the
cannellini beans and about ¼ cup of their liquid and stir to combine.

Add the broth and bring to a simmer. Reduce the heat to medium
to maintain a gentle simmer and cook for 5 minutes. Stir in the
escarole until it wilts, then cook for about 5 minutes, until tender.

Serve topped with a drizzle of olive oil and a sprinkle of fennel
pollen and cheese, if using.

NOTE ———————

*If using canned beans, drain and rinse
before adding, and add about ¼ cup water
to the pot.*

GREEN FRIED RICE

SERVES 4

So much of what makes food appetizing is texture, and I'm a sucker for just about anything with a good crunch. Repeatedly toasting the bottom layer of rice and stirring it back through the mixture gives this dish little crispy bits throughout! Here I've mixed the rice with Swiss chard, escarole, and baby kale, but you can use the same method for any sturdy greens you have on hand, such as kale or collards. This is one of the best reasons I can think of to keep cooked brown rice in your freezer.

2 tablespoons olive oil

2 tablespoons dark sesame oil

1 bunch of scallions, chopped

2-inch piece of ginger root, peeled and finely chopped

1 garlic clove, coarsely chopped

2 teaspoons kosher salt

2 cups cooked brown rice (page 94, preferably leftover)

1 bunch of Swiss chard, stems chopped fine and leaves cut into 1-inch pieces

1 bunch of escarole, chopped into 1-inch pieces

3 cups baby kale, chopped

1 avocado, sliced

Toasted sesame seeds, for garnish (optional)

Heat a large skillet over medium-high heat. Add the olive oil and 1 tablespoon of the sesame oil and heat for an additional minute. Add the scallions, ginger, garlic, and ½ teaspoon of the salt. Cook, stirring often, for about 2 minutes, until fragrant.

Add the rice and ½ teaspoon of the salt and toss to coat with the seasonings, then spread the mixture evenly over the bottom of the pan. Cook without stirring for 2 minutes. Using a wooden spoon, scrape the crispy rice from the bottom of the pan and stir well to distribute, then cook again without stirring for 2 minutes. Repeat these steps two more times to create layers of crispy, golden brown rice.

Add the Swiss chard stems and again cook without stirring for 2 minutes. Last, add the chard leaves, escarole, and kale along with the remaining tablespoon of sesame oil and 1 teaspoon salt. Stir in the greens a bit at a time; they will fit more easily as they wilt.

Cook until the greens are fully wilted and incorporated into the rice, 5 to 8 minutes. Serve topped with sliced avocado and, if desired, a sprinkling of toasted sesame seeds.

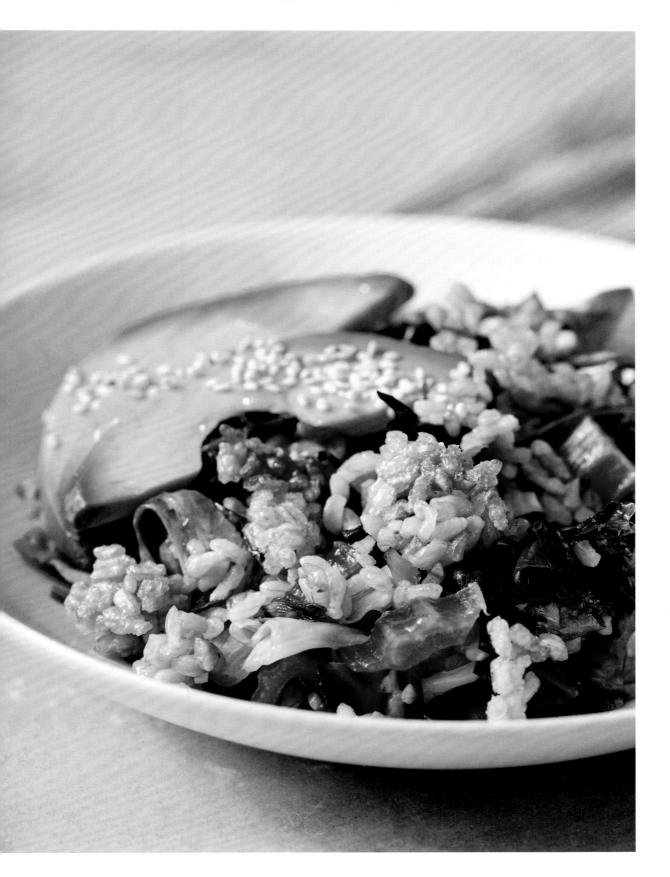

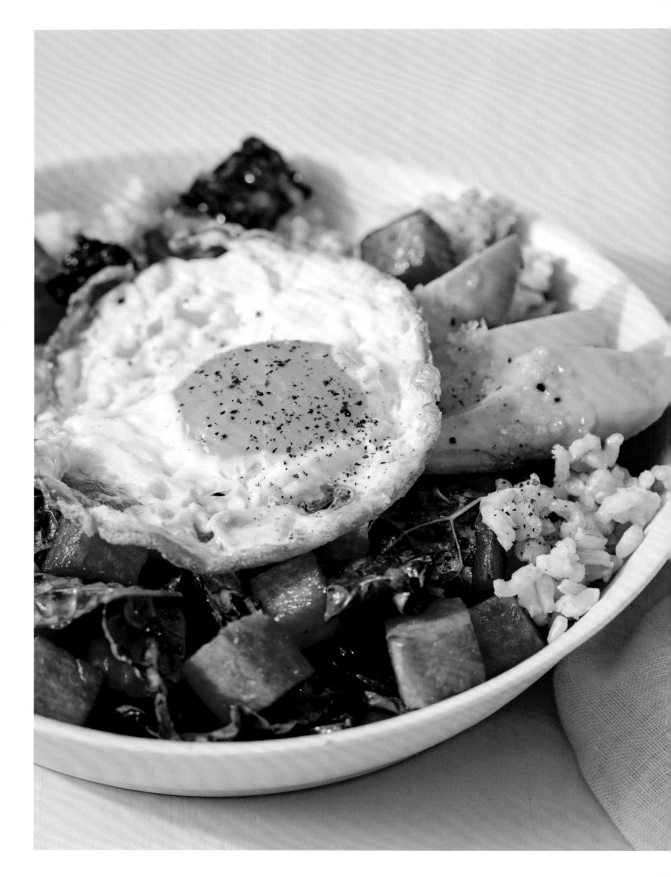

SPICED SWEET POTATO RICE BOWL WITH FRIED EGG

SERVES 2

This rice bowl is as colorful as it is packed with immunity-boosting antioxidants. I'd eat this for lunch or dinner, but if you like to start out with a hearty breakfast, it would be perfect for that too.

¼ cup olive oil, plus more to drizzle

1 small sweet potato, peeled and cut into ½-inch pieces

¾ teaspoon kosher salt

½ teaspoon ground turmeric

½ teaspoon ground cinnamon

2 cups chopped Tuscan kale

1 cup cooked brown rice (page 94), warmed

½ avocado, sliced

¼ teaspoon flake salt

2 large eggs (omit if using for a reboot meal)

Heat a medium skillet over medium heat. Add 2 tablespoons of the olive oil and heat for an additional minute. Add the sweet potato to the pan and season with ½ teaspoon of the salt. Cook, stirring often, for about 7 minutes, or until golden brown and just tender all the way through.

Sprinkle with the turmeric and cinnamon and cook for another minute to toast the spices. Add the kale to the pan along with another tablespoon of the olive oil. Cook, stirring often, for another 4 to 5 minutes, until the kale is wilted and beginning to brown.

Divide the brown rice between two bowls. Top each rice bowl with half the kale mixture. Fan half the avocado slices over each bowl and sprinkle the avocado with the flake salt.

Carefully wipe out the skillet with a paper towel and return to medium-high heat. Add the remaining tablespoon of oil and heat for another minute. Crack the eggs into the oil, being careful as they will pop and splatter a bit. Season each with ⅛ teaspoon kosher salt. Cook the eggs until the whites are just set and the edges are golden brown and crispy, about 2 minutes, spooning some of the oil in the pan over the yolks to help them set if needed. Slide an egg into each bowl. Drizzle with additional olive oil and serve.

STEAMED COD WITH COCONUT BROTH

SERVES 4

If a dish can be light yet rich at the same time, this one strikes that balance with a velvety base of coconut milk. Poaching all but guarantees your fish will come out moist and flaky, without the oil spatters and lingering smells that can come with pan-frying. You could also serve this over a small scoop of jasmine or basmati rice if you haven't already had your grains for the day.

2 tablespoons olive oil

1½ tablespoons peeled and chopped fresh ginger

2 shallots, chopped

2 garlic cloves, chopped

1¾ teaspoons kosher salt

½ teaspoon anchovy paste

1 (13.5-ounce) can light coconut milk

1 cup chopped Tuscan kale (about 3 leaves)

4 skinless fillets of cod or other flaky white fish (about 5 ounces each)

1 serrano or Fresno chile, thinly sliced (optional)

1 tablespoon fresh lime juice, from ½ lime

1 cup mixed herbs, such as Thai basil leaves, Italian basil leaves, and cilantro leaves

Lime wedges, for serving (optional)

Heat a medium skillet over medium-high heat. Add the oil, ginger, shallots, and garlic to the pan. Season with ¾ teaspoon of the salt and cook, stirring often, for about 3 minutes, or until fragrant. Stir in the anchovy paste and cook, stirring constantly, for 30 seconds. Stir in the coconut milk and bring to a simmer, then reduce the heat to medium-low to maintain a gentle simmer.

Add the kale to the coconut broth and stir to wilt slightly. Season the fish with the remaining teaspoon of salt and slide the fillets into the broth. Sprinkle with the sliced chile, if using. Cover the pan and poach for 8 minutes, or until the fish is cooked through and opaque. Squeeze the lime juice over the top.

To serve, use a slotted spatula to transfer each piece of fish to a shallow bowl and ladle a bit of broth and vegetables around it. Top each portion with some of the herbs. Serve with lime wedges, if desired.

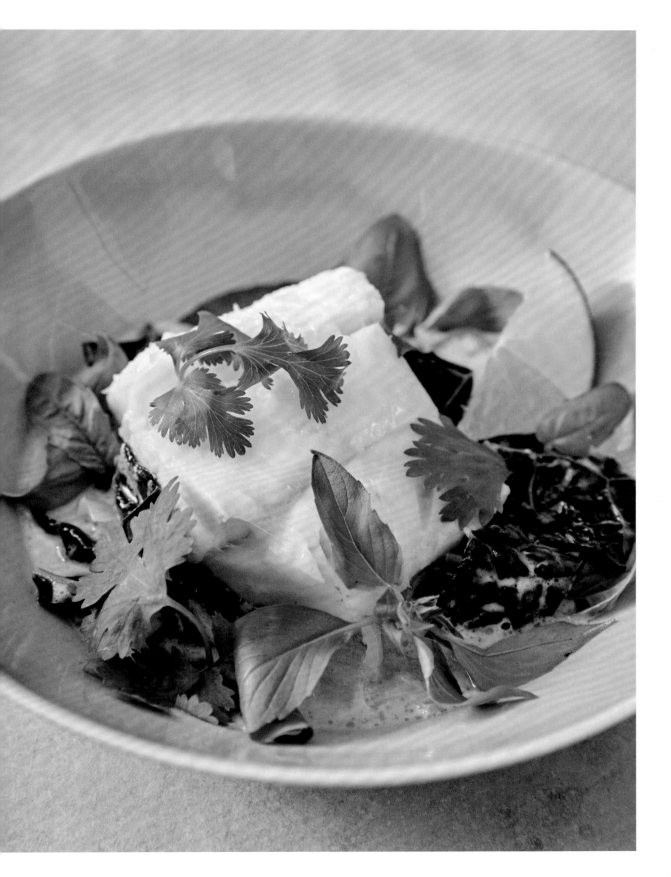

CHAPTER 11

Substantial Salads

One of the easiest ways to make sure you are getting plenty of vegetables and greens in your life is to plan one major meal a day around a salad. I am very happy with a main course salad, like those in this chapter, for dinner because I like to eat light later in the day (so I'm not going to bed on a heavy meal). But if salads sound more like lunch to you, that's just fine too.

Just about all of these salads can stand on their own as a one-dish meal; some, like the Millet Tabbouleh Salad (page 155), could be made more substantial by adding some leftover grilled protein like pounded chicken breasts (page 99). Leftovers make great pack-and-go lunches or sides to accompany a simple piece of grilled fish or meat. All of them are fresh and bright, just the thing for a special lunch or a dinner on the lighter side.

BROILED SALMON *and* FENNEL SALAD

SERVES 4

It's hard to believe something so elegant can be put together in under fifteen minutes, but it's true! Broiling is one of my favorite ways to cook fish because it's easy and fast, and I don't end up with grease splattered all over my stovetop. Make the dressing while the fish cooks, toss the veggies together, and when the salmon comes out of the oven, you're done.

1 pound salmon fillet, preferably wild king salmon, or Arctic char

1¾ teaspoon kosher salt

1 tablespoon olive oil

1 teaspoon Dijon mustard

1 tablespoon cider vinegar

2 tablespoons extra-virgin olive oil

4 cups baby arugula (about half of a 5-ounce container)

3 small inner celery stalks with pale leaves, chopped

1 large fennel bulb, stalks removed, very thinly sliced

½ cup torn fresh basil leaves

¼ teaspoon kosher salt

3 radishes, thinly sliced

Preheat the broiler to high and set an oven rack in the top third of the oven, or 6 to 7 inches below the heat source. Line a rimmed baking sheet with aluminum foil.

Place the salmon on the baking sheet. Season it with 1 teaspoon of the salt and drizzle evenly with the olive oil. Broil on high for 5 to 10 minutes, depending on the thickness of the salmon. The fish should be just light golden brown and flake easily but still be moist inside. Let cool slightly.

While it's still warm to the touch, use a fork to flake the fish into large pieces. The skin will stay on the pan, making it easy to break the flesh apart. Scrape off and discard any very dark flesh from the bottom of the fillet if desired.

Whisk together the mustard, vinegar, extra-virgin olive oil, and ½ teaspoon salt in a large bowl. Add the arugula, celery, fennel, and basil. Using your hands, toss gently to coat. Season with the remaining ¼ teaspoon salt and toss one more time. Divide the salad among four serving bowls. Top evenly with the radishes and chunks of flaked salmon.

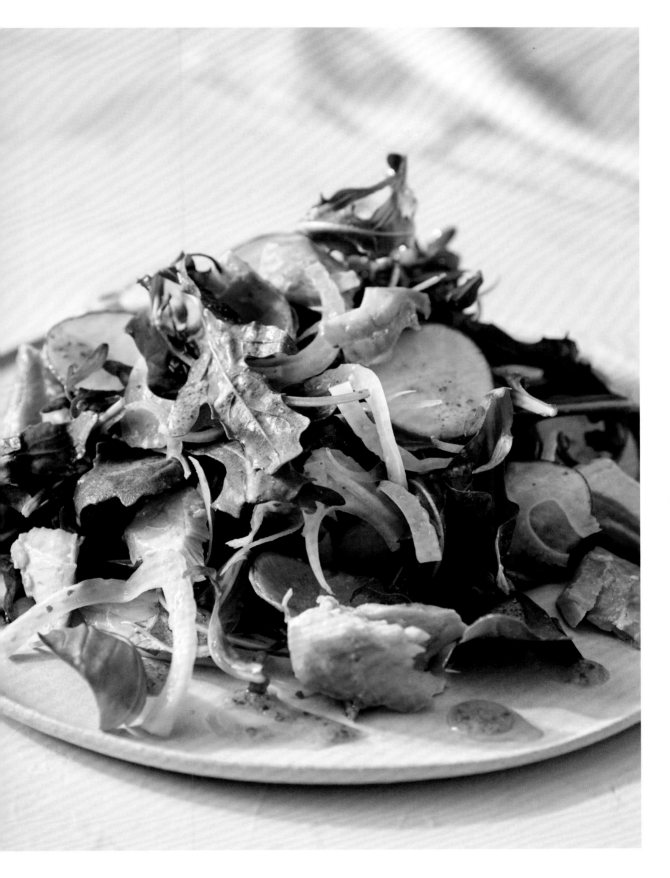

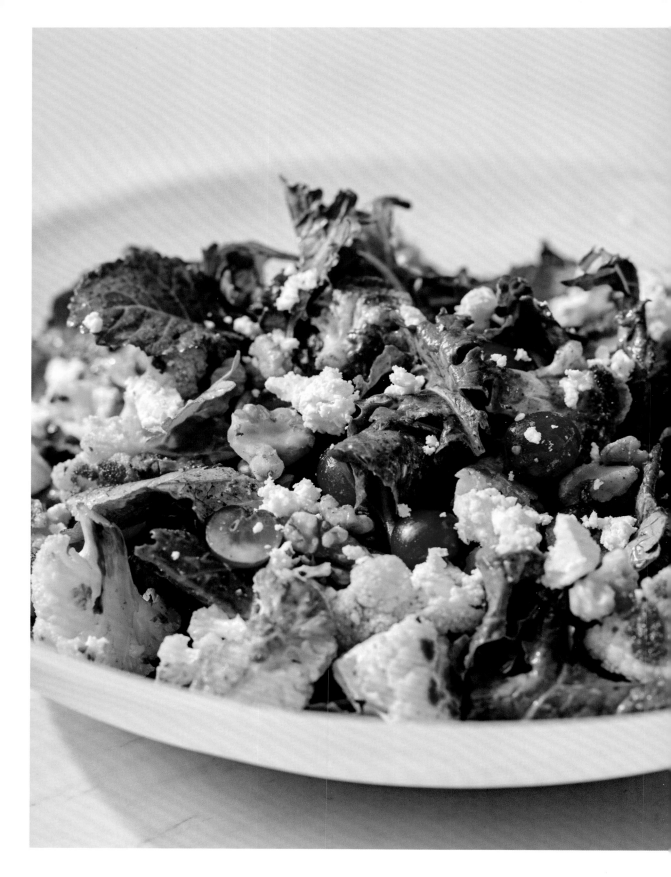

ROASTED CAULIFLOWER
and BABY KALE SALAD

SERVES 4

Cauliflower is having a movie-star moment. Everyone loves it for its versatility and ability to stand in for starchier veggies, but I'm constantly looking for new ways to infuse it with more flavor. Here, I give it a bit of a Middle Eastern spin with a salty-sweet blend of grapes and feta, and a hit of za'atar in the dressing, which warms up the roasted vegetables. If you don't have za'atar, mix together a few pinches of dried herbs, sesame seeds, and cumin, or substitute whatever herb blend you have on hand, such as herbes de Provence or Italian seasoning.

FOR THE SALAD

1 head of cauliflower, cut into 1-inch florets

2 tablespoons olive oil

1 teaspoon kosher salt

1 (5-ounce) container baby kale

1 cup halved seedless red grapes

¾ cup chopped toasted walnuts (see Note, page 129)

½ cup crumbled feta cheese (omit if using for reboot)

FOR THE DRESSING

2 teaspoons Dijon mustard

2 tablespoons cider vinegar

3 tablespoons extra-virgin olive oil

¼ teaspoon kosher salt

2 teaspoons za'atar

Preheat the oven to 450°F.

On a rimmed baking sheet, toss together the cauliflower, olive oil, and ¾ teaspoon of the salt. Roast for about 25 minutes, turning the cauliflower pieces halfway through, until tender and golden brown. Allow to cool slightly on the pan.

Meanwhile, make the dressing: In a large bowl combine the Dijon mustard, vinegar, extra-virgin olive oil, salt, and za'atar.

Add the warm cauliflower to the bowl with the dressing and toss to coat well. Add the baby kale, grapes, walnuts, and the remaining ¼ teaspoon salt. Gently toss to combine. Top with the feta, if using, and serve.

TANGY ESCAROLE "NIÇOISE" SALAD

SERVES 4

Composed salads like this one remind me of my time in France when I was studying pastry (and eating a lot of salads to balance out all of the croissants and pastry cream!). Because I've had issues with mercury in my system, I no longer eat tuna (like most big fish, it often has high levels of mercury), but with so many strong flavors, eggs for protein, and the buttery richness of the olives, I don't even miss it in my take on the classic salad Niçoise. Traditionally the anchovies are arranged on top of each serving, but if you have an anchovy hater at the table, try mashing them and stirring them into the dressing instead. Their pungent salinity really livens up the neutral potatoes and eggs.

FOR THE DRESSING

2 tablespoons whole-grain mustard

2 tablespoons extra-virgin olive oil

1 tablespoon cider vinegar

½ teaspoon kosher salt

FOR THE SALAD

4 baby Yukon Gold potatoes (omit if using for a reboot meal)

¼ pound trimmed green beans

½ cup mixed pitted olives, halved

1 head of escarole or 4 Little Gems, trimmed and chopped

¼ teaspoon kosher salt

4 hard-boiled eggs, halved

4 anchovy fillets (optional)

Freshly ground black pepper

Crumbled goat cheese (optional)

In a large bowl, whisk together the mustard, olive oil, vinegar, and salt until combined. Put 2 tablespoons of the dressing in a separate bowl.

To a saucepan, add the potatoes and cover with cold water. Set over high heat and bring to a boil. Reduce the heat to maintain a simmer and season well with salt. Boil for 5 minutes, then add the green beans. Cook 3 minutes longer, or until the potatoes are just tender when pierced with a knife. Drain well. Halve the warm potatoes and add them to the bowl with the 2 tablespoons dressing. Toss well to coat and let cool to room temperature. Once cool, add the green beans and olives and toss well to coat.

Meanwhile, add the escarole and ¼ teaspoon salt to the large bowl with the remaining dressing. Toss well to coat. Divide the escarole among four plates and divide the dressed vegetables among the greens. Top each salad with 2 egg halves, 1 anchovy (if using), a grind of black pepper, and some goat cheese, if using.

MILLET
TABBOULEH SALAD

SERVES 2 AS AN ENTRÉE OR 4 AS A SIDE

Millet is similar to quinoa, with small grains that cook up fluffy and separate, and like quinoa, it is a good source of protein as well as numerous minerals and vitamins. It's a great alternative to quinoa and brown rice if you've gotten into a bit of a grain rut. Here millet serves as a gluten-free alternative to bulgur wheat; it makes for a lighter, more refreshing tabbouleh. I also add strawberries, which, though quite nontraditional, provide a bit of sweetness and a pretty pop of color. To make it an even more substantial entrée salad, add bits of chicken or salmon. Of course, you can also serve it as a side to a simple summer meal.

1 cup raw millet

1 cup chopped flat-leaf parsley (about 1 large bunch)

⅓ cup chopped fresh mint leaves

1 shallot, chopped fine and rinsed under cold water

½ cup peeled and diced English cucumber

½ cup chopped strawberries

1½ teaspoons kosher salt

Juice of 1 lemon

⅓ cup extra-virgin olive oil

Baby arugula, baby spinach, or baby kale (optional)

Place the millet in a saucepan with 2 cups lightly salted water and bring to a boil over medium heat. Cover the pan, reduce the heat to low, and simmer the millet for 20 minutes. Remove from the heat and let stand for 10 minutes, then fluff with a fork. Let cool.

Place 1 cup of the cooked millet in a medium bowl and reserve the rest for another use (cooked millet can be frozen for up to 2 months). Add the parsley, mint, shallot, cucumber, and strawberries. Season with the salt, lemon juice, and olive oil. Mix well to coat evenly. Serve over greens, if desired.

GRILLED WEDGE SALAD

SERVES 4

Here I've transformed a steakhouse staple into a sophisticated warm side. Grilling changes the flavor and texture of radicchio, softening its sharp bite. Top it with a creamy, herby dressing and crisp, crunchy romaine, and people can't get enough. I make this year-round with a grill pan, but if you already have the barbecue grill fired up, you can char the radicchio directly on the grill grates. Gorgonzola dolce, which is a little sweeter and creamier than regular Gorgonzola, adds a special touch.

FOR THE DRESSING

1 tablespoon extra-virgin olive oil

½ cup plain low-fat Greek yogurt

1 teaspoon cider vinegar

¼ teaspoon onion powder

½ teaspoon garlic powder

⅛ teaspoon cayenne pepper

½ teaspoon kosher salt

1 tablespoon chopped fresh dill

FOR THE SALAD

1 head of radicchio

2 tablespoons olive oil

¼ teaspoon kosher salt

2 small heads of romaine

½ cup smoked almonds, chopped

⅓ cup crumbled Gorgonzola dolce

In a medium bowl, whisk together the extra-virgin olive oil, yogurt, and vinegar with 2 teaspoons water. Add the onion powder, garlic powder, cayenne, salt, and dill and mix well. Transfer to a jar and refrigerate for 1 hour to let the flavors mingle.

Preheat a grill pan over medium-high heat.

Cut the radicchio into 8 wedges and drizzle with the olive oil and sprinkle with the salt. Place the wedges on the grill and cook for 2 minutes per side, or until slightly browned and wilted.

Quarter the romaine lengthwise and arrange the wedges on a serving platter. Nestle the radicchio in between. Dollop the dressing over the top and scatter the smoked almonds and Gorgonzola over the top.

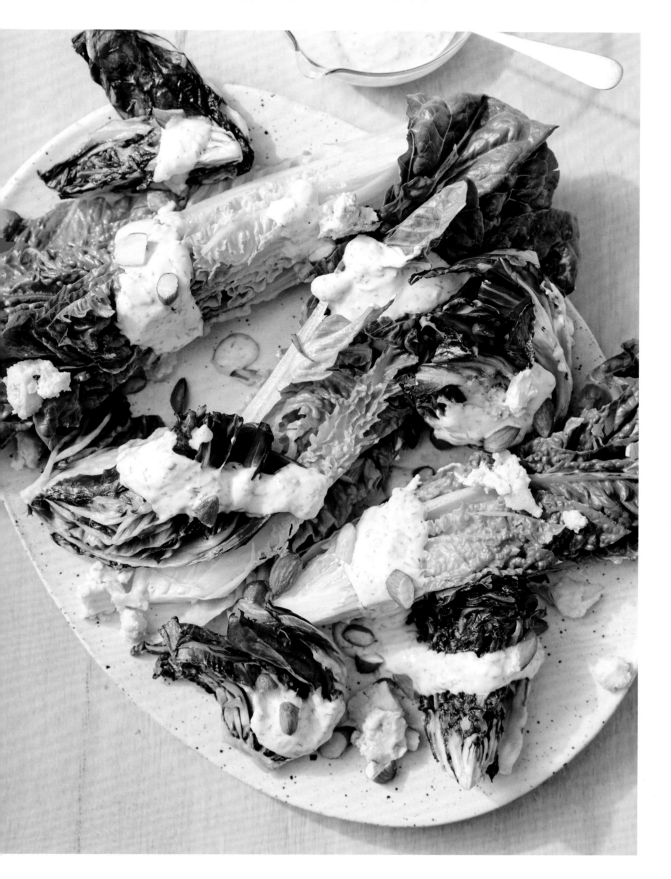

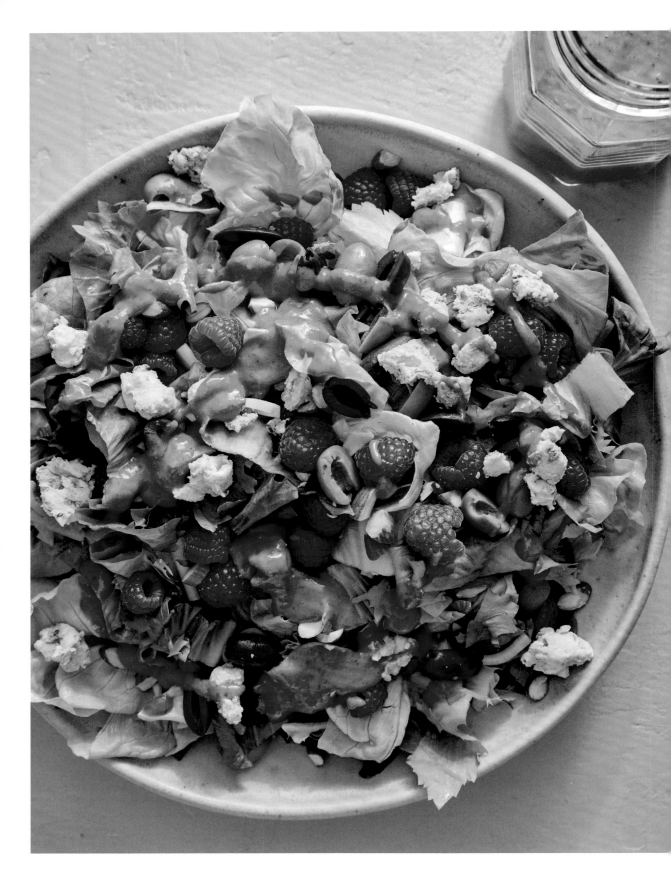

ESCAROLE *and* OLIVE SALAD WITH RASPBERRY DRESSING

SERVES 4

I've had many requests for this dressing recipe, especially from friends who have trouble getting their kids to eat salad. A full cup of raspberries blended into the dressing makes it bright pink and a bit tangy-sweet, so just about anything you put it on is instantly appealing. In the summer when raspberries are in season, I make it in big batches to keep in the fridge, then serve it on fish or chicken, or with veggies as a dip. It will keep for about a week.

FOR THE DRESSING

1 cup fresh raspberries

1 tablespoon Dijon mustard

1 tablespoon cider vinegar

3 tablespoons extra-virgin olive oil

¼ teaspoon kosher salt

FOR THE SALAD

1 small head of Bibb lettuce, chopped

1 small head of escarole, cut into 1-inch pieces

1 fennel bulb, stalks removed, thinly sliced

½ teaspoon kosher salt

1 cup pitted mixed olives, coarsely chopped

½ cup roasted almonds, coarsely chopped

¾ cup fresh raspberries

½ cup crumbled Gorgonzola dolce (optional; omit if using for a reboot meal)

For the dressing, combine the raspberries, mustard, vinegar, olive oil, and salt in a blender. Puree on high for about 1 minute, scraping down the sides halfway through, until emulsified. Set aside.

In a large bowl, toss together the lettuce, escarole, fennel, and salt. Begin by adding half the dressing and tossing well to coat. Taste the salad to determine if it needs more dressing. Depending on the size of your lettuces, you may not need to use all the dressing. Divide the salad among four bowls and top with the olives, almonds, and raspberries. Finish with the crumbled Gorgonzola, if using.

STEAK SALAD
WITH WHITE BEANS *and*
SWEET SHALLOT DRESSING

SERVES 4

Honestly, who doesn't like a steak salad? It's about the easiest thing there is to make and it's a true crowd-pleaser. In this version I've paired cannellinis with a relatively modest portion of beef, and the effect is almost like steak-and-potatoes in salad form. The warm steak wilts the greens slightly, and it's all bathed in a shallot-mustard dressing—irresistible! If you cook this outside over a gas or charcoal fire, the timing would be the same; just don't cook the meat with the lid down.

FOR THE STEAK

1 pound skirt steak

1½ teaspoons kosher salt

1 teaspoon olive oil

FOR THE DRESSING

2 shallots, sliced into thin rings

3 tablespoons olive oil

½ teaspoon kosher salt

1 tablespoon Dijon mustard

2 tablespoons cider vinegar

FOR THE SALAD

1 cup cooked cannellini beans (page 90)

4 radishes, thinly sliced

3 tablespoons chopped fresh tarragon

1 small head of escarole or romaine, cut into 1-inch pieces

Ten minutes before cooking, take the steak out of the refrigerator. Heat a grill pan over medium-high heat. Dry the meat well with paper towels and season with the salt. Drizzle it with the olive oil, place it on the grill pan, and top with a heavy pan or an aluminum foil-covered brick to ensure it makes contact with the hot ridges. Cook the steak without moving it for about 4 minutes, until a deep golden crust has formed. Flip the steak and cook for an additional 4 minutes. Transfer the steak to a plate to rest for at least 10 minutes.

Meanwhile, in a small skillet, combine the shallots, olive oil, and salt. Place over medium heat and cook for about 3 minutes, until the shallots are soft and fragrant. Remove from the heat and allow to cool in the pan for 5 minutes.

Transfer the shallots to a large bowl and whisk in the mustard and vinegar until the dressing is emulsified. Add the cannellini beans, radishes, tarragon, and escarole and toss to coat with the dressing. Thinly slice the rested steak against the grain and add it to the salad. Toss one more time and serve.

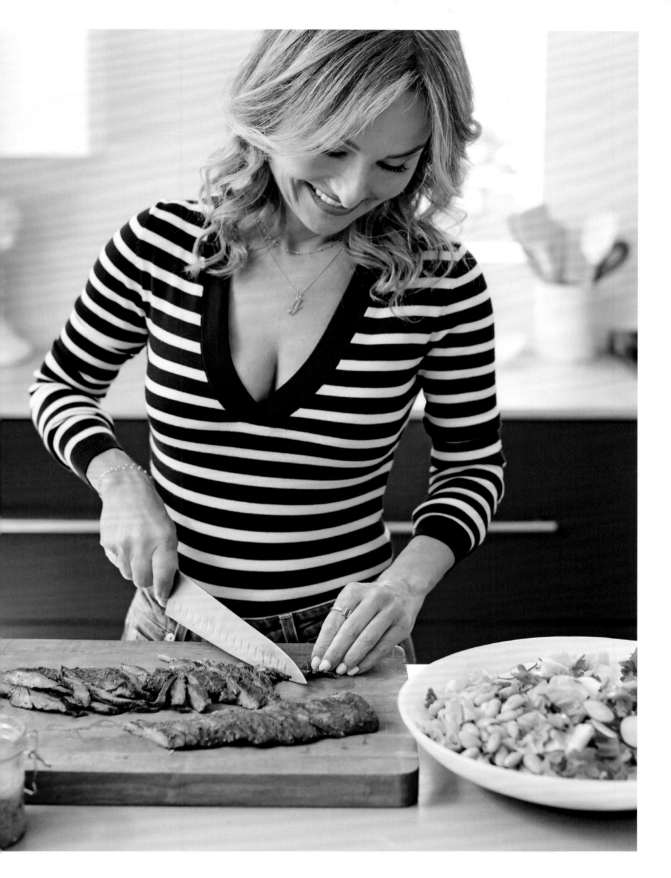

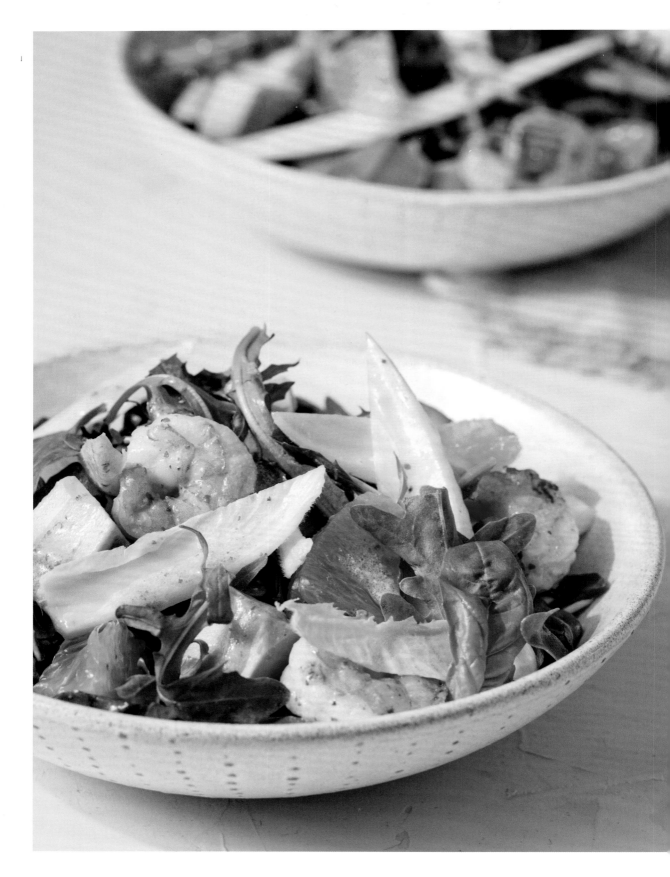

SHRIMP *and* ENDIVE SALAD

SERVES 4

The combo of arugula, orange, and endive is one I eat all the time as a side salad; adding shrimp turns this into a meal, and a really pretty one at that. Once the shrimp are cooked, this is super-duper easy. You could also toss in ½ cup of cooked quinoa or brown rice if you want to give the salad a little more heft.

FOR THE SHRIMP

1 tablespoon olive oil

16 large shrimp (just over ½ pound), peeled and deveined

½ teaspoon kosher salt

FOR THE SALAD

1 tablespoon whole-grain mustard

2 tablespoons fresh lemon juice, from 1 lemon

3 tablespoons extra-virgin olive oil

¾ teaspoon kosher salt

2 Belgian endives, sliced lengthwise into 1-inch strips

4 cups baby arugula

1 orange, segmented

1 avocado, diced

¼ cup torn fresh basil leaves

Heat the olive oil in a large skillet over medium-high heat. Add the shrimp and spread them in an even layer. (This can be done in two batches if your skillet isn't large enough to allow each shrimp to make contact with the hot surface.) Season the shrimp with ½ teaspoon salt and cook without moving them for 2 minutes, or until they are bright pink and beginning to brown a bit on the undersides. Flip and cook 1 to 2 minutes longer, or until the shrimp are opaque all the way through. Set aside to cool slightly.

In a large bowl, whisk together the mustard, lemon juice, extra-virgin olive oil, and ½ teaspoon of the salt. Add the shrimp to the dressing and toss to coat. Divide the shrimp among four serving plates, leaving the dressing in the bowl. Add the endive, arugula, orange segments, avocado, basil, and the remaining ¼ teaspoon salt to the dressing in the bowl and toss well. Top the shrimp with the salad and serve.

RED, WHITE,
and BLUE SALAD

Wally's is a great wine bar and restaurant with a couple of locations in LA. They serve a salad similar to this one, and I order it every single time, it's just that good. What sets this salad apart are the stunning colors of the ingredients and the quick-pickle topping, which adds a touch of acidity. If you can find an aged Gorgonzola, also called Gorgonzola picante, use that here. It's a little sharper and drier than younger blues.

FOR THE QUICK PICKLE

1 tablespoon sugar

¼ cup champagne vinegar

1 teaspoon kosher salt

½ English cucumber, peeled and diced (about 1 cup)

FOR THE SALAD

1 tablespoon champagne vinegar

1 teaspoon whole-grain mustard

3 tablespoons extra-virgin olive oil

½ teaspoon kosher salt

2 heads of radicchio, chopped

1 head of curly endive or frisée, chopped

1½ cups red grapes, halved

1 cup blueberries

½ cup chopped roasted and lightly salted pistachios

½ cup crumbled Gorgonzola Piccante

In a small saucepan, combine the sugar, vinegar, ¼ cup water, and the salt. Bring to a simmer over medium heat. Remove from the heat and allow to cool for 5 minutes. Place the cucumber in a small bowl. Pour the brine over the cucumbers and let sit at room temperature for 30 minutes.

Meanwhile, in a large bowl, whisk together the vinegar, mustard, olive oil, and salt. Add the radicchio, endive, grapes, and blueberries. Toss well to coat. Drain the cucumber and sprinkle it over the top along with the pistachios and Gorgonzola. Toss one last time and serve.

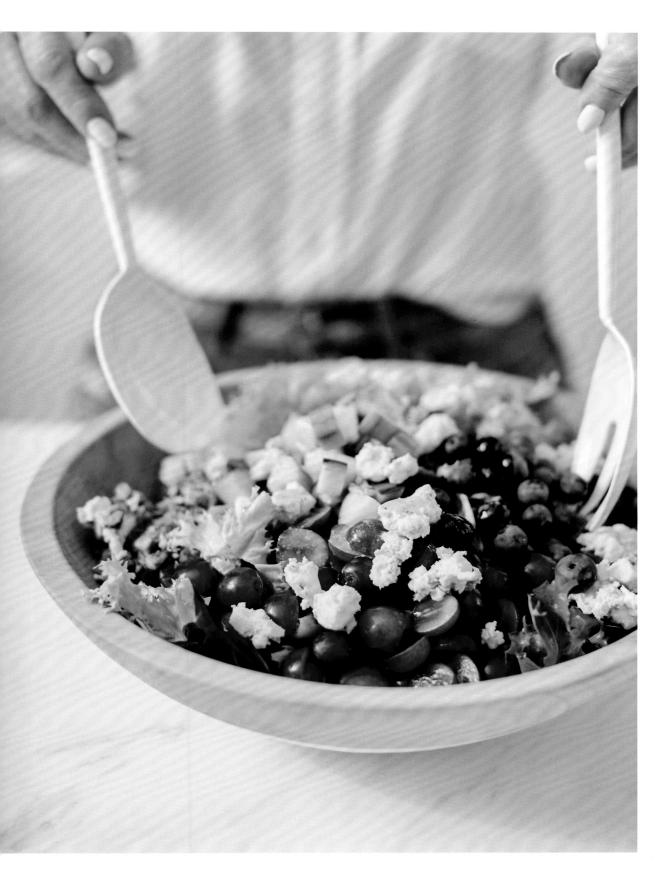

CHAPTER 12

Pastas

One of the things I'm asked about most often is what to make for dinner when you're trying to eat less meat, something that has become a priority for a lot of people. Pasta and grain dishes like risotto are the obvious answers, even when you're trying to eat a little cleaner. As I've said, pasta isn't the enemy: it's about keeping everything in balance and in the right proportions.

The recipes in this section are satisfying but they won't sit heavily in your stomach the way so many cheesy, creamy, ultrarich pastas can—even vegetarian ones. In fact, these are not necessarily vegan or vegetarian at all—you will find small amounts of dairy, chicken broth, or eggs used here and there to add body and richness. But none of them put animal products at the center—just bold flavors and lots of veggie goodness. If you need to avoid gluten, use your favorite gluten-free pasta; just remember you need to rinse and drain the pasta after cooking to keep it from getting gummy. Whichever kind of pasta you use, the smaller portion sizes here—just 2 or 3 ounces instead of the usual 4 ounces (or more)—won't send your carb intake for the day into the red zone.

SPAGHETTI WITH ROSEMARY
AND LEMON 169

FUSILLI WITH PESTO AND
GREEN BEANS 170

SPAGHETTI WITH SHRIMP AND ARUGULA 172

HEARTY CHICKEN BOLOGNESE
WITH ZUCCHINI NOODLES 173

BEYOND BOLOGNESE
WITH PENNE 175

PACCHERI WITH MUSHROOMS
AND PISTACHIOS 176

FUSILLI WITH CHICKEN
AND BROCCOLI RABE 179

CAMPANELLE WITH SALMON
PUTTANESCA 180

PENNE WITH SPICY CALABRIAN SHRIMP 183

ARTICHOKE AND BRUSSELS SPROUT
BROWN RICE RISOTTO 184

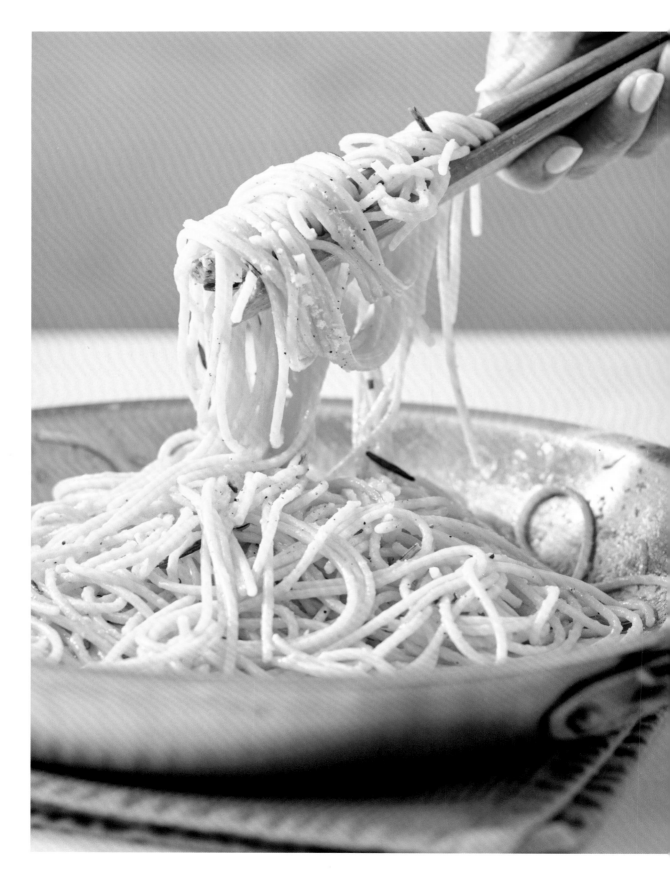

SPAGHETTI WITH ROSEMARY *and* LEMON

SERVES 6

Pasta doesn't have to be complicated to be luscious. This dish is very simple but flavorful, so even a smaller portion makes a nice, light meal when paired with a big green salad. You could also add bits of cooked asparagus, broccoli, zucchini—even shrimp if you're not going for a meatless main.

1 pound regular or gluten-free spaghetti

¼ cup olive oil

3 garlic cloves, smashed and peeled

3 fresh rosemary sprigs

½ teaspoon kosher salt

1 teaspoon grated lemon zest

1 cup freshly grated pecorino Romano cheese, plus more for garnish

½ teaspoon freshly ground black pepper, plus more to taste

Bring a large pot of water to a boil over high heat. Season the water generously with kosher salt. Add the pasta and cook for 1 minute less than directed on the package, usually 6 to 7 minutes. Reserve 1½ cups of the pasta cooking water, then drain the pasta well. If using gluten-free pasta, rinse under cool running water and drain again.

Heat a large skillet over medium-high heat. Add the oil and heat for another minute. Add the garlic and rosemary and fry for 2 to 3 minutes, until the rosemary is fragrant and crispy. Transfer the rosemary to a paper-towel-lined plate to drain. Continue to cook the garlic until golden brown. Using a slotted spoon, remove and discard the garlic.

Add the cooked pasta to the skillet and, before combining with the oil in the pan, sprinkle the bare pasta with the salt, lemon zest, and cheese. Add ½ cup of the reserved pasta water and begin tossing to coat the pasta in the light cheese sauce. Continue to toss, adding more pasta water as needed to create a creamy sauce. Season with the black pepper and serve topped with additional cheese, crispy rosemary needles, and more black pepper, if desired.

FUSILLI WITH PESTO
and GREEN BEANS

SERVES 4

Pairing pesto with two kinds of veggies makes this one of the greenest pasta dishes you can have, and if Jade is any example, it's one kids are happy to eat. The pesto coats each twist of pasta like a velvety jacket, making every bite fun to eat. You'll have leftover pesto; refrigerate it for up to a week.

¼ cup pine nuts

2 cups fresh basil leaves

1 garlic clove

1½ teaspoons kosher salt, plus more to taste

¼ teaspoon freshly ground black pepper, plus more to taste

Approximately ⅔ cup extra-virgin olive oil

1 cup grated Parmigiano-Reggiano

1 (8-ounce) package whole-grain or gluten-free fusilli

2 tablespoons olive oil

1 shallot, chopped

½ pound green beans, trimmed and cut into 1-inch pieces

1 (10-ounce) bag frozen peas

½ cup ricotta cheese

In a small, dry skillet, toast the pine nuts over medium heat until fragrant and just beginning to brown, 3 to 4 minutes. Transfer to a plate to cool.

In a food processor, combine the basil, garlic, ½ teaspoon of the salt, ¼ teaspoon pepper, and the pine nuts. Pulse until finely chopped. With the machine running, gradually add enough of the extra-virgin olive oil to form a smooth and thick paste; you may not need it all. Transfer the pesto to a medium bowl and stir in ½ cup of the cheese. Season with more salt and pepper to taste. Measure out ⅓ cup of the pesto and save the rest for another time.

Bring a large pot of water to a boil over high heat. Season the water generously with kosher salt. Add the pasta and cook 1 minute less than directed on the package, about 5 minutes. Reserve ⅓ cup of the pasta cooking water, then drain the pasta well. If using gluten-free pasta, rinse it under cool running water and drain again.

While the pasta cooks, heat a large skillet over medium-high heat. Add the olive oil and shallot to the pan with ½ teaspoon of the salt and cook for 1 minute. Add the green beans and the remaining ½ teaspoon salt. Cook, stirring often, for about 4 minutes, or until the beans are just cooked through. Stir in the peas and cook for another minute.

Add the drained pasta to the pan along with the reserved pasta water. Sprinkle the pasta with the remaining ½ cup cheese, add ⅓ cup of the pesto, and toss well to coat. Serve with a dollop of ricotta on top.

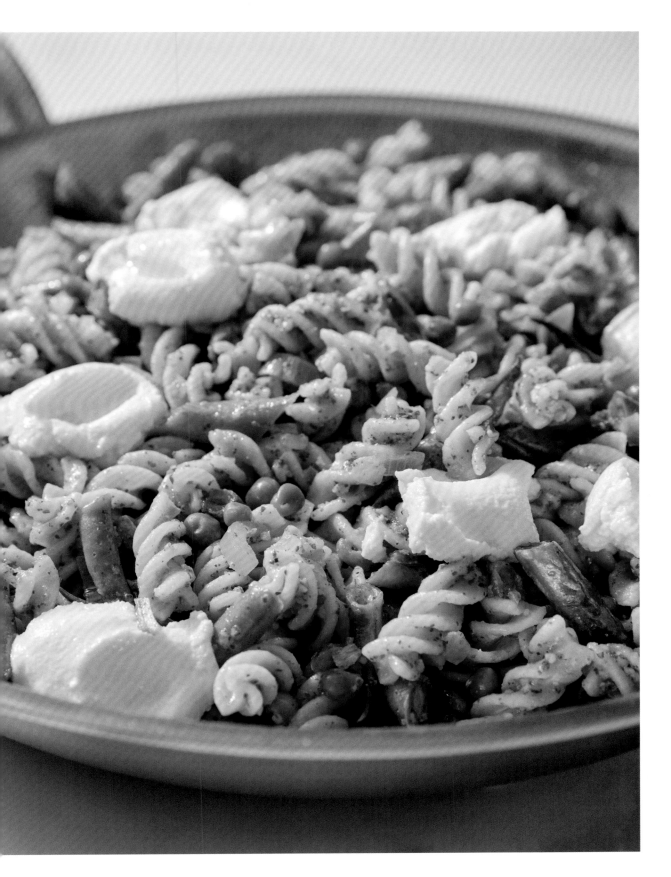

SPAGHETTI WITH SHRIMP
and ARUGULA

SERVES 4

I first had this seafood sauce as a topping for homemade Sardinian gnocchi, which is a real treat but also, it has to be said, something of a project. Pairing it with dried pasta puts it squarely in the weeknight wheelhouse, especially if you have frozen shrimp on hand. It has the familiar flavors of a scampi but with a healthy spin, thanks to the addition of arugula and the option of going gluten-free.

½ pound regular or gluten-free spaghetti

3 tablespoons olive oil

2 garlic cloves, smashed and peeled

1 pound medium shrimp, peeled and deveined

1 teaspoon kosher salt

½ teaspoon crushed red pepper flakes

½ cup dry white wine

½ cup freshly grated Parmigiano-Reggiano, plus more for serving

½ (5-ounce) container baby arugula (about 4 cups), roughly chopped

1 teaspoon grated lemon zest

Bring a large pot of water to a boil over high heat. Season the water generously with kosher salt. Add the pasta and cook for 2 minutes less than directed on the package, about 6 minutes. Reserve ½ cup of the pasta cooking water, then drain the pasta well. If using gluten-free pasta, rinse it under cool running water and drain again.

While the pasta cooks, heat a large skillet over medium-high heat. Add the oil and garlic and cook for 2 minutes, or until fragrant. Add the shrimp, ½ teaspoon of the salt, and the red pepper flakes. Cook, stirring often, for about 2 minutes, or until the shrimp are pink and almost completely opaque. Add the wine to the pan and stir with a wooden spoon to loosen any browned bits. Season with the remaining ½ teaspoon salt. Simmer for about 2 minutes, until the shrimp are just opaque all the way through and the sauce has reduced slightly.

Add the pasta to the skillet and, before combining, sprinkle with the cheese. Add the arugula and lemon zest and toss until well combined and the arugula is wilted. Add some of the reserved pasta water as needed to maintain a sauce. Serve topped with additional cheese if you like.

HEARTY CHICKEN BOLOGNESE WITH ZUCCHINI NOODLES

SERVES 6

Spiralized noodles of zucchini, known in some quarters as zoodles, do a great job of standing in for pasta, but paired with a mild sauce they can taste a bit watery and bland. No such problem here! The only way I can describe this Bolognese is gutsy, with a deeper, heartier base of red wine and tomato puree that I've amped up even further with a bit of anchovy and red pepper flakes. It's incredibly satisfying and bold, yet light at the same time, and even a generous portion won't sit heavily on your stomach.

2 tablespoons olive oil

1 pound ground chicken

1½ teaspoons kosher salt

1 small red onion, chopped

1 medium carrot, finely chopped

3 garlic cloves, finely chopped

1 teaspoon anchovy paste

¼ teaspoon dried oregano

½ teaspoon red pepper flakes

1 cup dry red wine

1 (28-ounce) can pureed tomatoes

1 (3-inch) piece of Parmesan rind

2 fresh basil stems, plus ¼ cup chopped basil

1 pound zucchini noodles

1 cup freshly grated Parmigiano-Reggiano, plus more for serving (optional)

Extra-virgin olive oil, for drizzling

Heat a medium Dutch oven over medium-high heat. Add the olive oil and chicken and cook until the meat is lightly browned, about 5 minutes, breaking it into very small pieces with a wooden spoon. Season with ½ teaspoon of the salt. Add the onion, carrot, garlic, anchovy paste, oregano, and red pepper flakes and stir to combine. Season with an additional ½ teaspoon of the salt and cook for 3 more minutes, or until the vegetables are soft and fragrant.

Stir in the red wine, using the wooden spoon to scrape up the brown bits from the bottom of the pan. Simmer until the liquid has almost completely cooked down, about 5 minutes. Stir in the tomato puree and season with the remaining ½ teaspoon salt. Nestle the Parmesan rind and basil stems into the sauce. Reduce the heat to medium and simmer the sauce for 25 minutes, uncovered, stirring occasionally.

Fish the Parmesan rind and basil stems out of the sauce and discard, then add the zucchini noodles to the sauce. Sprinkle with the cheese, if using, then toss to coat with the sauce. Cook for 2 minutes, or until the zucchini noodles are just crisp tender. Serve, drizzling each portion with a little extra-virgin olive oil and sprinkling with the chopped basil and a little more cheese, if you like.

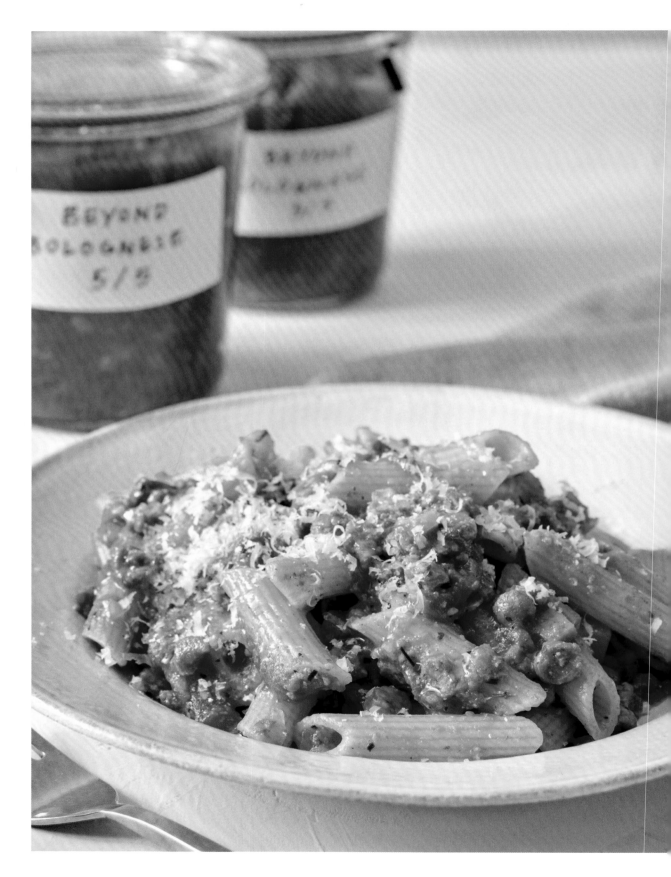

BEYOND BOLOGNESE
WITH PENNE

SERVES 6 WITH LEFTOVER SAUCE

Each and every time I announce I'm making Bolognese pasta for dinner, I get a happy reaction from my family. So when I thought about how to incorporate some plant-based meat products into our weekly meal rotation, it made sense to use them in a recipe I know is a universal crowd-pleaser. This is a lighter version than the classic, which is made with beef and pork and simmered with milk, but it provides just as much decadent flavor. I always make it in big batches and freeze the extra sauce for emergency weeknight meals.

2 tablespoons olive oil

1 pound plant-based "ground meat," such as Beyond Meat, thawed if frozen

½ red onion, chopped

1 medium carrot, finely chopped

2 garlic cloves, smashed and peeled

1 cup dry white wine

1 (28-ounce) can whole San Marzano tomatoes, crushed by hand

1 (3-inch) piece of Parmesan rind (optional)

2 fresh whole basil stems

½ teaspoon kosher salt

1 pound penne, regular or gluten-free

1 cup freshly grated Parmigiano-Reggiano, plus more for serving

Extra-virgin olive oil, for drizzling

Heat a medium Dutch oven over medium-high heat. Add the olive oil and the "ground meat," breaking it into very small pieces with a wooden spoon. Cook until the crumbles are lightly browned, about 5 minutes. Add the red onion, carrot, and garlic to the pan and stir to combine. Cook for 3 minutes, or until the vegetables are soft and fragrant.

Add the white wine, scraping up the brown bits from the bottom of the pan with the wooden spoon. Simmer for 5 minutes, or until the wine is almost completely reduced. Stir in the tomatoes. Nestle the cheese rind, if using, and basil stems into the sauce and add the salt. Reduce the heat to medium and simmer the sauce, stirring occasionally, for 25 minutes.

Meanwhile, bring a large pot of water to a boil over high heat. Season generously with kosher salt. Add the pasta to the water and cook until the pasta is still quite al dente, about 2 minutes less than directed, about 6 minutes. Reserve 1 cup of the pasta cooking water. Drain the pasta well and rinse under cool water; drain again. Remove the basil stems and cheese rind from the sauce and discard, then add the pasta to the sauce. Sprinkle the cheese directly onto the bare pasta, then toss the pasta well to coat with the sauce, thinning as needed with the reserved pasta water. Serve drizzled with extra-virgin olive oil and sprinkled with additional cheese, if desired.

PACCHERI WITH MUSHROOMS
and PISTACHIOS

SERVES 6

Mushrooms with Marsala and pistachios is a fantastic combination of flavors, which is why this pasta is currently one of my faves. I think it looks especially dramatic with paccheri, a large tubular pasta that resembles sliced calamari, but any short cut shape would work here too. Try using royal trumpet mushrooms, morels, cremini, shiitakes, or oyster mushrooms. They all have different flavors and textures, and experimenting with new varieties is part of the fun!

3 tablespoons olive oil

2 garlic cloves, smashed
and peeled

1 pound assorted
mushrooms, sliced
¼ inch thick

¾ teaspoon kosher salt

1 shallot, chopped

¼ cup sweet Marsala

½ cup low-sodium chicken
broth

2 tablespoons unsalted
butter

1 pound paccheri pasta or
gluten-free penne

1½ cups freshly grated
Parmigiano-Reggiano

2 cups baby arugula

½ cup salted roasted
pistachios, chopped

Bring a large pot of water to a boil over high heat.

Heat a large skillet over medium-high heat. Add 2 tablespoons of the oil and heat for 30 seconds. Add the garlic and mushrooms to the pan. Season with the salt and stir. Cook the mushrooms without stirring again for about 4 minutes, or until the mushrooms on the bottom are golden brown. Stir, then repeat this sequence until the mushrooms are browned and cooked through, about 10 minutes longer.

Add the remaining tablespoon of oil and the shallot and cook for 2 minutes, stirring often. Add the wine and, using a wooden spoon, loosen any browned bits from the bottom of the pan. Simmer for 1 minute, or until almost entirely cooked down. Add the chicken broth and butter and simmer for 3 minutes to emulsify and thicken slightly.

When the water boils, season it generously with kosher salt. Add the pasta and cook for 2 minutes less than directed on the package, about 10 minutes, until not quite al dente. Using a mesh skimmer or tongs, transfer the pasta directly from the pot into the sauce. Add ⅓ cup of the pasta cooking water to the pan. Sprinkle the bare pasta with 1 cup of the cheese. Toss well to combine and coat in the sauce. Simmer over medium heat for 2 minutes, tossing often, to finish the pasta, adding more cooking water as needed to make a light sauce. Stir in the arugula and heat until just wilted; add the remaining cheese. Sprinkle with the pistachios and serve.

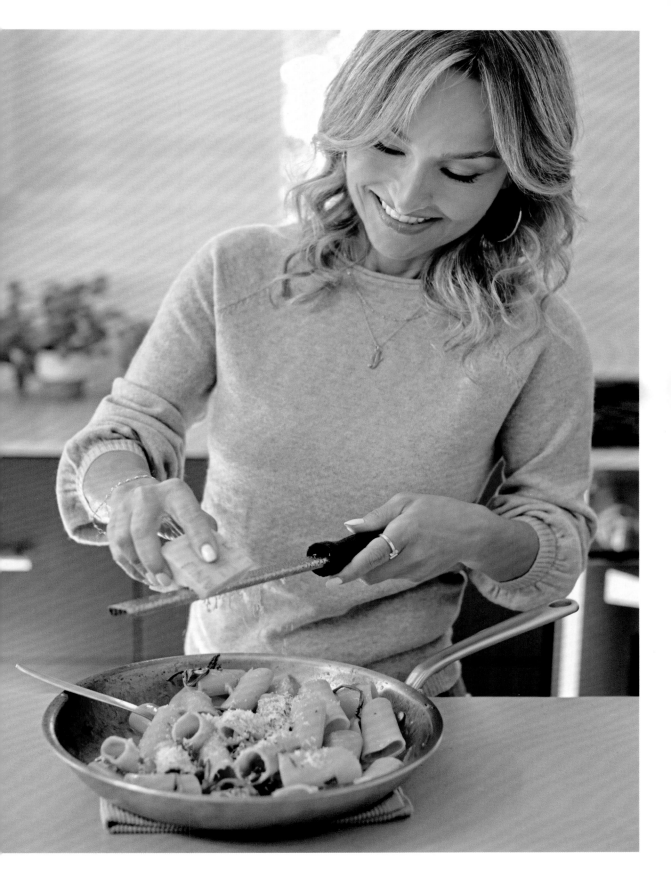

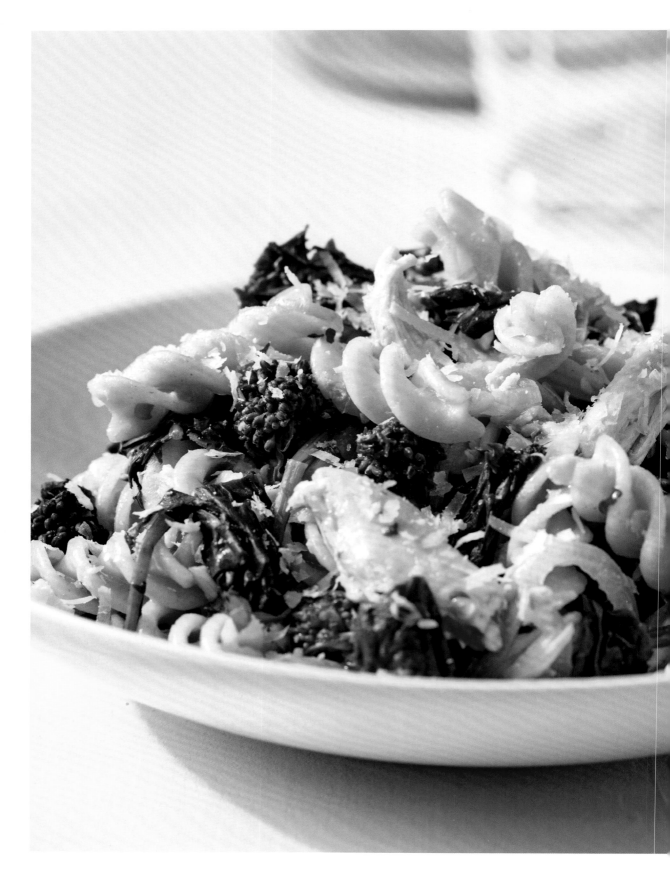

FUSILLI WITH CHICKEN
and BROCCOLI RABE

SERVES 4

Pastas that work as a one-dish meal are real weeknight wins, and this one definitely qualifies. With almost equal amounts of chicken and pasta, it's a lighter update on the classic pairing of sausage and broccoli rabe. Using pre-cooked chicken makes this so fast to pull together!

1 bunch of broccoli rabe, cut into 1-inch pieces

½ pound regular or gluten-free fusilli

3 tablespoons olive oil

2 garlic cloves, sliced

1 shallot, sliced

1 teaspoon kosher salt

½ teaspoon crushed red pepper flakes (optional)

2 cups shredded cooked chicken (page 99) or about half of a rotisserie chicken, shredded

½ cup freshly grated Parmigiano-Reggiano, plus more for serving

Bring a large pot of water to a boil over high heat. Season the water generously with kosher salt. Blanch the broccoli rabe for 1 minute, then use a wire skimmer to transfer it to a colander to drain. Add the pasta to the same water and cook for 2 minutes less than directed on the package, 4 to 6 minutes. Reserve ½ cup of the pasta cooking water, then drain the pasta well. If using gluten-free pasta, rinse it well under cool running water, then drain again.

While the pasta cooks, heat a large skillet over medium-high heat. Add the oil and heat for a minute. To the hot oil, add the garlic, shallot, ½ teaspoon of the salt, and the red pepper flakes. Cook, stirring often with a wooden spoon, for 2 minutes, or until soft and fragrant. Add the chicken and toss well to coat in all the flavors. Add the broccoli rabe and the remaining ½ teaspoon salt and cook until the greens begin to wilt, about 2 minutes. Carefully stir the mixture and cook for another 2 minutes, or until the broccoli rabe is completely wilted and almost cooked through.

Add the pasta and the Parmigiano. Toss well to combine, adding some of the reserved pasta water as needed to create a light sauce. Serve with additional cheese at the table.

CAMPANELLE WITH SALMON PUTTANESCA

SERVES 6

Canned tuna is the usual anchor for puttanesca sauce, but when I tried this version at a seaside trattoria on Capri, it made me see that tried-and-true dish in a whole new light. Made with fresh salmon, it's much lighter and brighter, but no less flavorful. Plus it's a good way to stretch half a pound of salmon to feed a group! You could also make it with clams or shrimp.

1 pound campanelle pasta, gluten-free if desired

¼ cup plus 2 tablespoons olive oil, plus more to drizzle

½ teaspoon kosher salt

½ pound boneless, skinless salmon fillet, cut into 1-inch cubes

1 red onion, halved and thinly sliced

2 garlic cloves, chopped

1 pound cherry tomatoes (about 1½ pints), halved

½ cup dry white wine, such as Pinot Grigio

1½ cups mixed pitted olives, halved if large

2 teaspoons fresh oregano leaves, chopped

¾ cup fresh flat-leaf parsley leaves, chopped

1 cup freshly grated Parmigiano-Reggiano, plus more for serving

Bring a large pot of water to a boil. Season the water generously with kosher salt. Add the pasta and cook for 2 minutes less than directed on the package, about 5 minutes. Reserve ½ cup of the pasta cooking water, then drain the pasta. If using gluten-free pasta, rinse it well under cool running water, then drain again.

While the pasta cooks, heat a large skillet over medium-high heat. Add 2 tablespoons of the olive oil. Season the salmon evenly with ¼ teaspoon of the salt and place in the hot pan. Cook the fish cubes without moving them for 2 to 3 minutes, or until golden brown on the first side. Add the onion and garlic and cook, stirring often, for another minute.

Add the tomatoes and season with the remaining ¼ teaspoon salt. Cook the tomatoes, stirring often, for another 3 minutes, or until beginning to soften. By this point the salmon will be flaking apart a bit, but try to keep it in larger pieces to prevent it from drying out too much. Reduce the heat to medium and stir in the white wine, scraping the pan to loosen any brown bits. Simmer for 2 minutes to reduce slightly, then stir in the olives, oregano, and parsley.

Add the pasta to the pan and sprinkle with the cheese. Toss to coat. Add ¼ cup of the reserved pasta cooking water and the remaining ¼ cup olive oil and toss to combine. Add more pasta water as needed to create a silky sauce. Serve with additional cheese and olive oil, if desired.

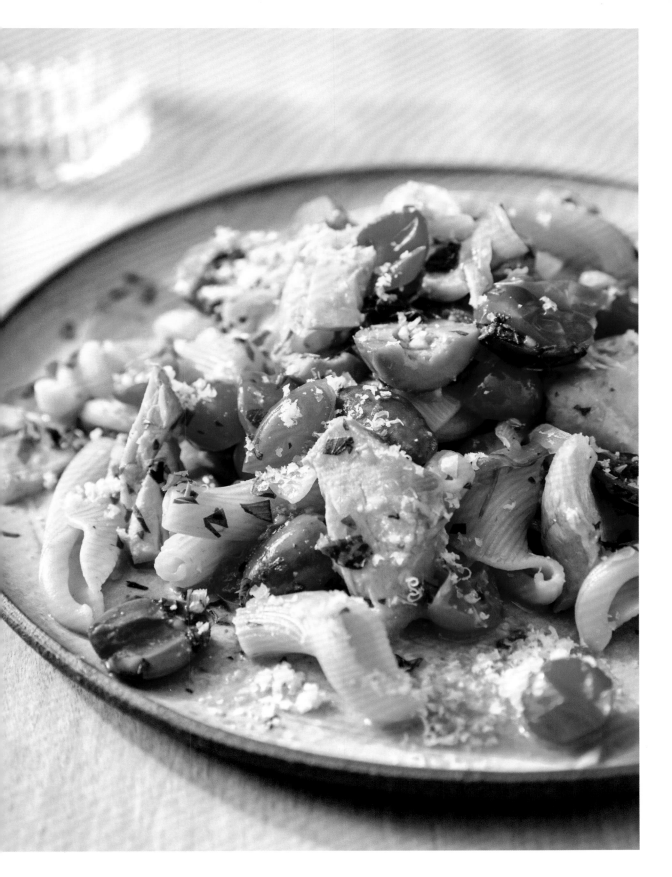

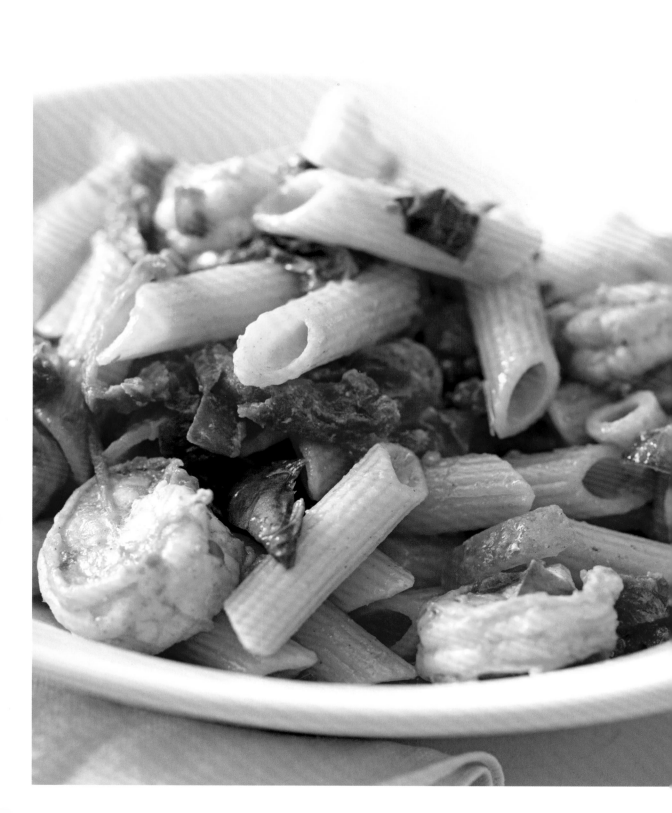

PENNE WITH SPICY CALABRIAN SHRIMP

SERVES 4

I use Calabrian chile paste the way other people use sriracha, by which I mean in just about everything that needs a little extra kick. In this case it turns what could be a pretty standard pantry dinner into a really sexy entrée. If your skillet is not large enough to hold all the shrimp in a single layer, cook them in two batches.

1 pound large shrimp, peeled and deveined

1 teaspoon grated lemon zest

2 garlic cloves, smashed and peeled

1½ teaspoons Calabrian chile paste

3 tablespoons olive oil, plus more to drizzle

¾ teaspoon kosher salt

1 tablespoon fresh lemon juice, from ½ lemon

½ pound regular or gluten-free penne

½ red onion, diced

½ cup chopped marinated sun-dried tomatoes

½ cup freshly grated Parmigiano-Reggiano, plus more for serving

¼ cup chopped fresh basil

In a medium bowl, combine the shrimp, lemon zest, garlic, chile paste, 2 tablespoons of the olive oil, ½ teaspoon of the salt, and the lemon juice. Toss well to coat in all the flavors. Set aside at room temperature for 10 minutes.

Bring a large pot of water to a boil. Season the water generously with kosher salt. Add the pasta and cook for 2 minutes less than directed on the package, about 6 minutes. Reserve ½ cup of the pasta cooking water, then drain the pasta. If using gluten-free pasta, rinse it under cool running water, then drain again.

Heat a large skillet over medium-high heat. Add the remaining tablespoon of olive oil along with the onion, the remaining ¼ teaspoon salt, and the sun-dried tomatoes. Cook for about 4 minutes, or until the onion is soft and fragrant, stirring often. Add the shrimp to the pan and spread them evenly so they all make contact with the bottom of the pan. Cook for 3 to 4 minutes, stirring often, until the shrimp are bright pink and opaque all the way through.

Add the drained pasta to the skillet and sprinkle with the cheese. Toss well to incorporate the cheese and coat the pasta with the flavored oil. Add the reserved pasta water and basil and toss again to create a sauce. Serve with more cheese and a drizzle of olive oil, if desired.

ARTICHOKE *and* BRUSSELS SPROUT BROWN RICE RISOTTO

SERVES 4 TO 6

A risotto can't be rushed, and that goes double when you're using brown rice, which takes a full hour to become nice and creamy. The artichokes cook along with the rice, breaking down a bit to infuse the dish with flavor, though you should still see a few intact leaves throughout. This is the perfect project for a lazy Sunday dinner when you can spend some time in the kitchen. I find it relaxing to stand and stir with a glass of wine, maybe listening to a podcast or doing some food prep for the upcoming week. Don't walk away as the rice simmers, though; it does need to be minded.

2 tablespoons olive oil

1 shallot, chopped

6 ounces frozen or canned artichoke hearts

1 cup short-grain brown rice

¾ teaspoon kosher salt

½ cup dry white wine

3¾ to 4 cups chicken broth, homemade (page 96) or low-sodium store-bought

10 ounces Brussels sprouts, thinly sliced

½ cup grated pecorino cheese, plus more to finish

Extra-virgin olive oil, for drizzling

Heat a Dutch oven over medium heat. Add the oil and shallot and cook, stirring often, for 2 minutes, or until softened. Add the artichokes and cook for another 5 minutes, or until starting to brown. Stir in the rice and salt and stir for about 3 minutes to coat the rice in the oil and toast it slightly. Add the white wine and cook until it is almost entirely absorbed, about 4 minutes, stirring often.

Add 1½ cups of the chicken broth and bring to a simmer. Cook, stirring often, for about 20 minutes, until almost all the liquid is absorbed. Add another 1¼ cups broth and continue to cook and stir for another 20 minutes. Finally, stir in the Brussels sprouts and 1 more cup of the broth and cook just until the rice is cooked through and the risotto is creamy, another 10 to 15 minutes, stirring even more frequently. Stir in the pecorino and a touch more broth if needed to make it fluid and creamy. Serve drizzled with extra-virgin olive oil and sprinkled with more pecorino, if desired.

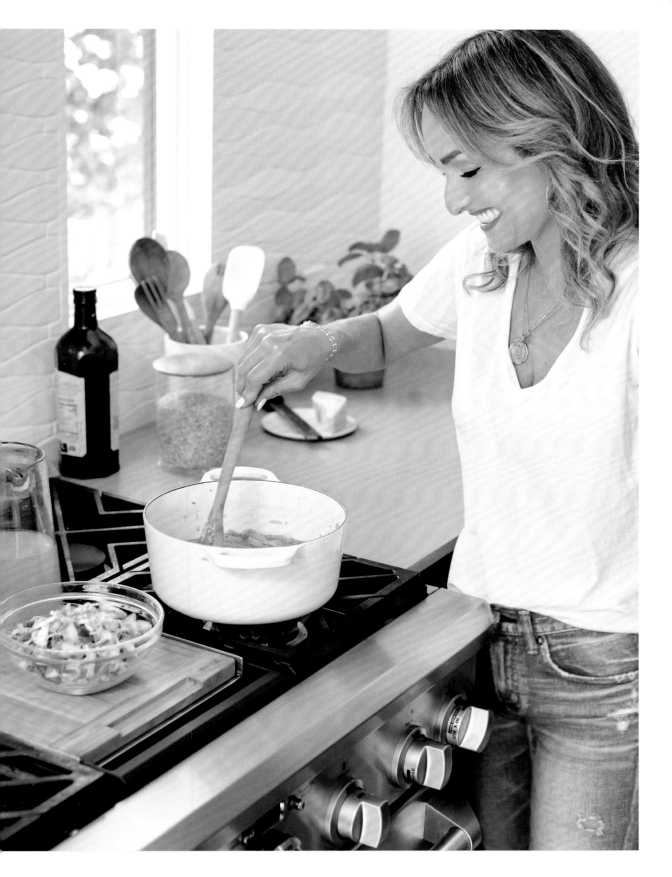

CHAPTER 13

Main Plates:
With and Without Meat

I'm not here to wade into the great debate over the merits of a meatless diet. There are strong feelings on both sides and equally strong arguments in favor of diets that avoid animal products and those that include them. I'm happy to say that if you are in the vegetarian or vegan camp, there are a *ton* of recipes in this book that will make your day—even a couple in this chapter! For those who eat fish and meat, the recipes here are all designed to give you plenty of protein satisfaction even though the portions themselves are quite moderate.

You'll notice that there are a lot of options for lean, clean proteins like chicken and fish, and relatively fewer suggestions for beef, lamb, and pork. That's a reflection of the way I tend to eat, saving things like a steak, chops, or hearty stew for the weekends and leaning toward lighter, cleaner options during the week. I've also begun incorporating plant-based meat substitutes into my meal plans now and then (check out the Bolognese recipe on page 175 as well as the stuffed peppers on page 206) for dishes with a mouthfeel similar to ground beef without the meat. If you have a passionate love affair with red meat, see if you can adopt a more long-distance relationship during the week. I know it really made a difference for me.

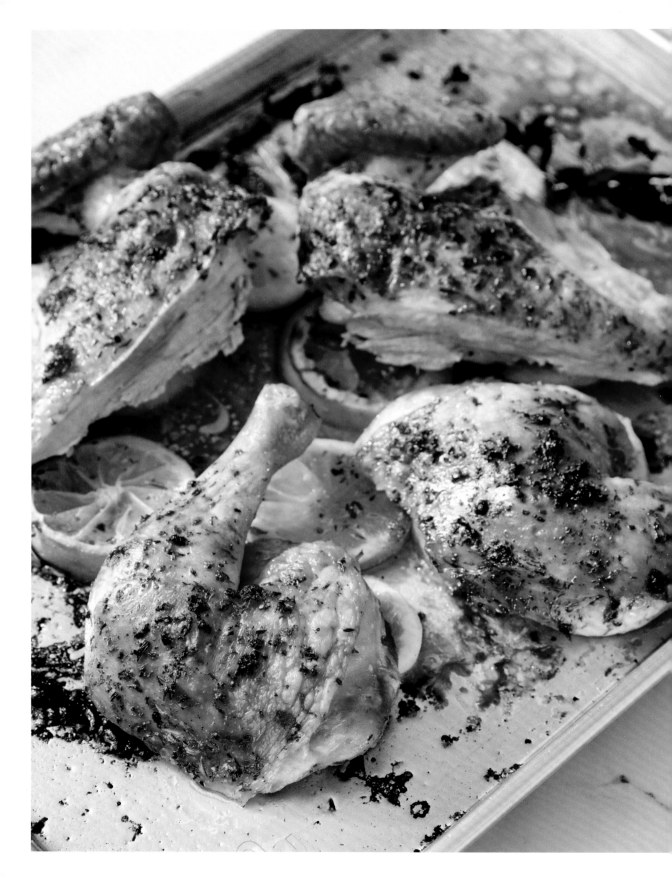

AMALFI LEMON CHICKEN

SERVES 2 TO 4

Lemon? Check. Crispy skin? The delicious smell of fresh herbs as the bird roasts? Easy enough to make on a weeknight? Check, check, and check again. This recipe ticks all the boxes for me, and I'm sure it will for you as well. Many markets now sell spatchcocked chickens that have had their backbones (and sometimes breastbones) removed, which allows the chicken to open up flat. My friends tell me they've made this using just breast and thigh pieces and it works fine that way too. I make this at least once a week.

4 tablespoons olive oil

3 large lemons, zested and sliced

2 teaspoons chopped fresh thyme leaves

1 teaspoon chopped fresh rosemary leaves

2½ teaspoons kosher salt

1 chicken (about 3½ pounds), backbone and breastbone removed

Preheat the oven to 450°F. Drizzle 2 tablespoons of the olive oil over a rimmed baking sheet. Arrange the lemon slices on the sheet to form a "rack" for the chicken.

In a small bowl, combine the lemon zest, thyme, rosemary, and salt. Sprinkle one-third of the salt rub on the flesh side of the chicken. Flip the chicken and rub the remaining salt mixture over and under the skin of the whole chicken. Lay the chicken skin side up on the bed of lemons and drizzle with the remaining 2 tablespoons olive oil. Roast for 40 to 45 minutes, basting every 15 minutes with the pan drippings, until golden brown and an instant-read thermometer inserted in the thigh reads 160°F. Transfer the chicken to a cutting board to rest for 10 minutes before carving.

Meanwhile, use a fork to mash the lemon pulp into the pan juices, discarding the rinds. Spoon the sauce over the chicken just before serving.

CHICKEN MILANESE

SERVES 4

Sure, this is a bit of a treat, but rice flour and gluten-free panko make it a little lighter and easier on the tummy. I serve it the way they do in Italy, topped with an arugula salad dressed with lemon and salt, or without the salad and just a squeeze of lemon juice.

4 chicken cutlets (about 4 ounces each)

1¾ teaspoons kosher salt

¼ cup rice flour

2 large eggs, beaten

¾ cup gluten-free panko

3 tablespoons olive oil

¼ teaspoon freshly ground black pepper (optional)

1 lemon, cut into wedges

Place the cutlets between two pieces of plastic wrap. Using the smooth side of a meat mallet or the back of a small skillet, gently pound the cutlets until very thin and of even thickness.

Season the cutlets evenly on both sides with ½ teaspoon of the salt. Place the flour, eggs, and panko in three separate shallow bowls. Season the flour with ¼ teaspoon of the salt, the eggs with ¼ teaspoon of the salt, and the panko with ½ teaspoon of the salt. One at a time, dredge the seasoned chicken cutlets first in the flour, then the egg mixture, and last the panko, pressing gently to make sure the chicken is evenly coated with the crumbs.

Heat a large skillet over medium heat until hot. Add the oil to the hot pan and heat for another 10 seconds. Working in batches, add the breaded chicken to the pan and cook for 4 to 5 minutes, or until the first side is deep golden brown and the chicken begins to look cooked around the edges. Flip the cutlets and cook on the second side until golden brown and crispy, about 3 minutes longer. Transfer the chicken to a wire rack to drain briefly and season with the remaining ¼ teaspoon salt, plus black pepper, if desired. Serve hot with 1 or 2 lemon wedges apiece.

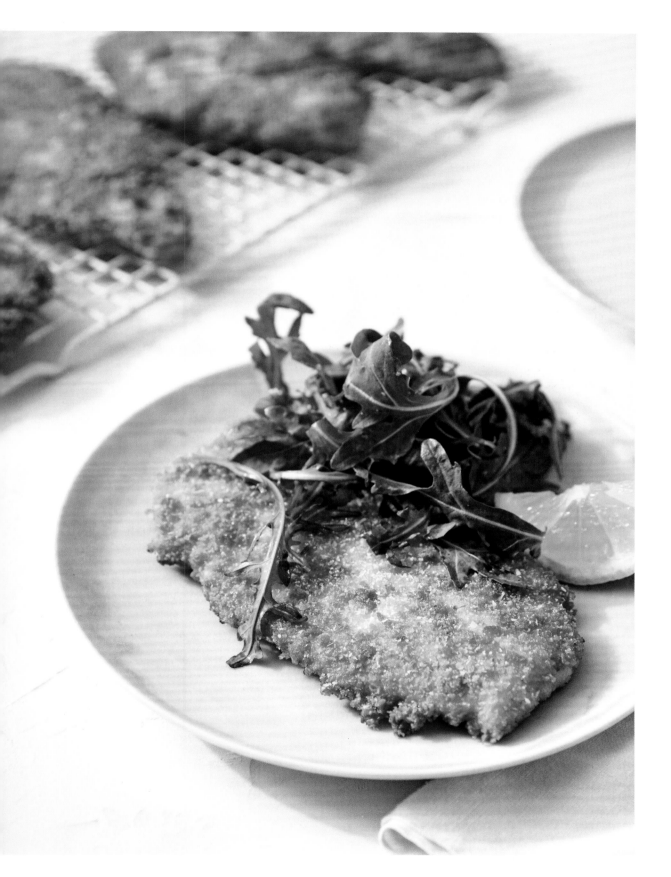

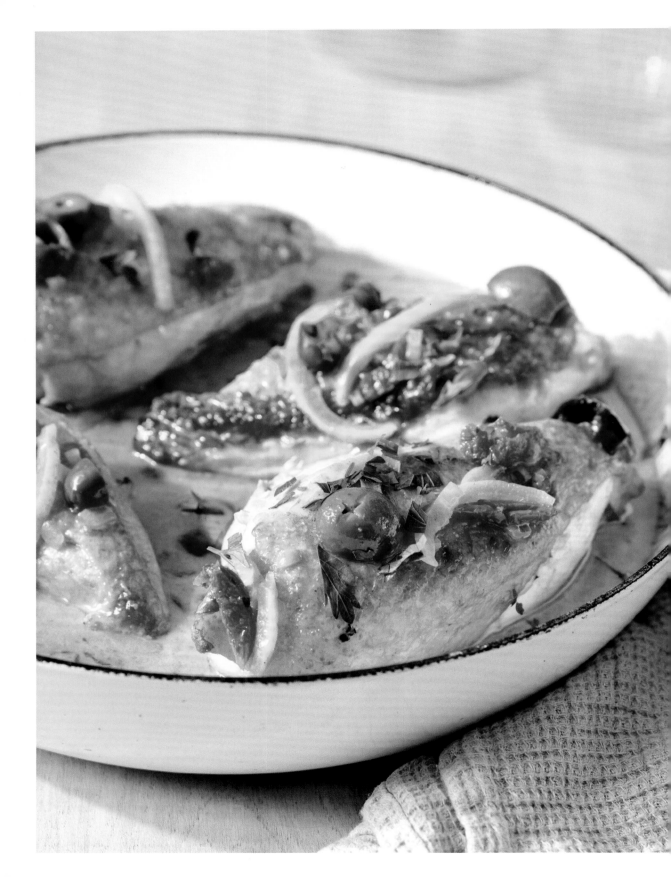

RAFFY'S CHICKEN · WITH PRESERVED LEMONS

SERVES 4

Like everyone else, I'm always looking for new ways to serve chicken, and this saucy dish, made with preserved lemons, is a winner. My aunt Raffy turned me on to preserved lemons, a specialty of Moroccan cooking that she has been making at home for years. Nowadays they are easier to find in stores so you don't have to salt and brine your own the way she does (she also dehydrates sliced lemons for cocktails, but that's another story), and they are really worth seeking out if you've never tried them. Served over quinoa or brown rice, this is a great company dish.

2 tablespoons olive oil

4 bone-in, skin-on chicken breast halves

1¼ teaspoons kosher salt

1 shallot, chopped

1 preserved lemon, pulp discarded, thinly sliced (see Note)

½ cup pitted mixed marinated olives, halved

½ cup oil-packed sun-dried tomatoes, chopped

1 cup dry white wine

1 cup chicken broth, homemade (page 96) or low-sodium store-bought

4 fresh oregano sprigs

2 tablespoons chopped fresh flat-leaf parsley

NOTE ———

If you can't find preserved lemons, use a small lemon, seeded and cut into small bits.

Heat a medium straight-sided skillet over medium-high heat. Add the oil. Dry the chicken breasts well with paper towels and season them with the salt. Place the breasts skin side down in the hot pan and cook without moving them for 6 minutes, or until the skin is deep golden brown. Using tongs, flip the chicken skin side up and cook for another 5 minutes. Transfer to a plate.

To the same pan, add the shallot and cook over low heat, stirring occasionally, for 1 minute, or until softened. Add the preserved lemon, olives, and sun-dried tomatoes and stir to combine. Stir in the white wine, scraping up the brown bits from the bottom of the pan with a wooden spoon, and simmer for 3 minutes to reduce the sauce slightly.

Stir in the chicken broth and bring the liquid to a simmer over medium heat. Add the oregano and the chicken, spooning some of the liquid over the breasts. Cover the pan, reduce the heat to low, and simmer gently for 25 minutes, or until an instant-read thermometer inserted in the thickest part of the breast registers 160°F. Remove from the heat and allow the chicken to rest in the sauce for 10 minutes. Discard the oregano sprigs and stir in the parsley. Serve the chicken with plenty of the sauce.

EASY CHICKEN PICCATA

SERVES 4

This is a classic for a reason: it takes less than twenty minutes to prepare, uses ingredients straight from the pantry, and is pretty much universally enjoyed. What's not to love? Make sure the skillet you use has a metal handle that won't melt under the broiler, and be careful—it gets extremely hot!

4 boneless, skinless chicken breasts (about 6 ounces each)

1½ teaspoons kosher salt

1 teaspoon olive oil

1 teaspoon grated lemon zest

2 tablespoons fresh lemon juice, from 1 lemon

⅔ cup chicken broth, homemade (page 96) or low-sodium store-bought

2 tablespoons drained capers

2 tablespoons unsalted butter, at room temperature

2 tablespoons chopped fresh flat-leaf parsley

Position a rack in the top third of the oven and preheat the broiler.

Season the chicken breasts evenly with the salt and rub with the olive oil. Arrange them in an ovenproof skillet large enough to hold them without overlapping. Add the lemon zest and juice, chicken broth, and capers to the pan.

Place the pan under the broiler and cook the chicken for 10 to 12 minutes, until it is browned and the internal temperature reads 160°F on an instant-read thermometer when inserted into the thickest part of a breast. Transfer the chicken to a platter to rest.

Place the skillet on the stovetop and bring the broth to a simmer over medium heat. Add the butter and any juices that have accumulated around the chicken and whisk into the sauce until incorporated. Stir in the parsley. Slice the chicken and serve with the sauce spooned on top.

SOLE WITH
LEMON-CAPER SAUCE

SERVES 2 TO 4

If you have everything you need in the pantry—and of course you have capers, lemons, and Calabrian chile paste, right?—you just need to do is pick up some fish on the way home and this dinner is all but on the table. Thin lemon sole fillets are ideal for this recipe, as they cook in less than five minutes; if you use a thicker type of sole, or another fish, like snapper, you may need to cook it two or three minutes longer. Warm up some of the quinoa you've cooked ahead of time (see page 92) and drizzle the lemony sauce over all.

4 lemon sole fillets

1¼ teaspoons kosher salt

2 tablespoons extra-virgin olive oil

3 tablespoons unsalted butter, at room temperature

⅓ cup rice flour, for dredging

1 garlic clove, minced

¼ cup drained capers, rinsed

¼ cup fresh lemon juice, from 1½ lemons

½ cup chicken broth, homemade (page 96) or low-sodium store-bought

½ teaspoon Calabrian chile paste or crushed red pepper flakes

½ teaspoon chopped fresh oregano

2 tablespoons chopped fresh flat-leaf parsley

Using paper towels, dry the sole fillets very well. Season them on both sides with 1 teaspoon of the salt. Place a medium skillet over high heat. When it's hot, put 1 tablespoon of the olive oil and 1 tablespoon of the butter in the pan. When the butter is fully melted and the bubbles have subsided, dredge two of the fillets in the rice flour, coating both sides. Shake off the excess and add the fish to the pan. Reduce the heat to medium-high. Cook for 2 to 3 minutes on the first side, or until beginning to brown around the edges. Using a wide spatula, gently flip the fish and cook the second side for 30 seconds. Transfer the fillets to a plate. Repeat the process with the remaining tablespoon of olive oil, another tablespoon of butter, and the last two fish fillets.

When all four fillets are cooked, add the garlic and capers to the empty pan and stir over medium heat for about 15 seconds, until fragrant. Add the lemon juice and chicken broth and stir, scraping up the bits from the bottom of the pan. Season with the remaining ¼ teaspoon salt. Simmer for about 2 minutes to reduce the liquid slightly. Finish the sauce by stirring in the remaining tablespoon of butter, the chile paste, and oregano. Spoon the sauce over the fish, sprinkle with the parsley, and serve.

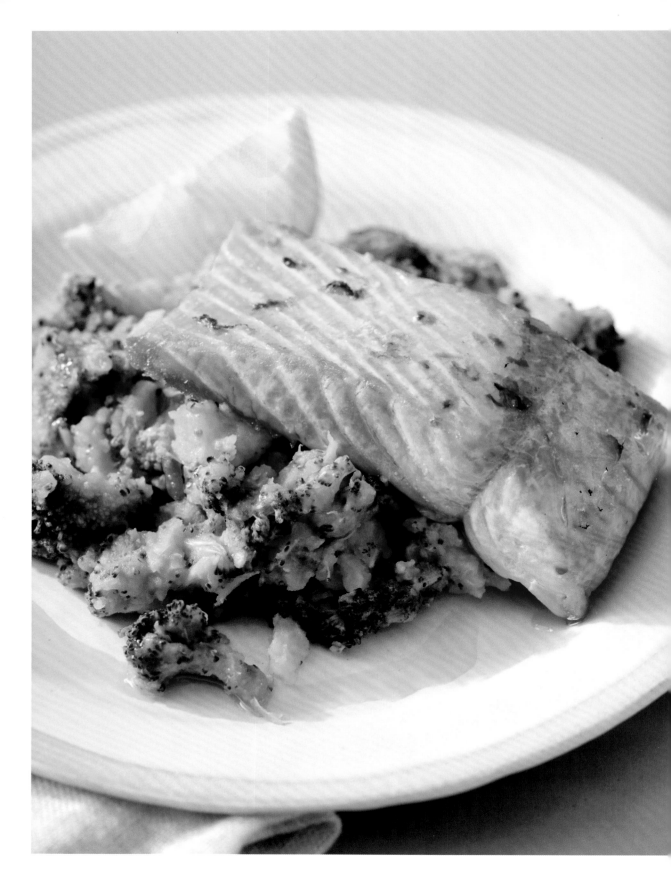

BROILED SALMON WITH CRUSHED BROCCOLI

SERVES 4

Depending on how good you are at multitasking, you can have this dinner ready in about twenty minutes, maybe twenty-five if you throw in a nice big salad. Crushing the broccoli and potato together makes a bright green bed for the fish, and while it has the soothing, homey qualities of mashed potatoes, it is really more greens than carbs. Win-win!

FOR THE MASH

1 Yukon Gold potato (about 8 ounces), peeled and cut into 1-inch pieces

2 broccoli crowns (about 1 pound total), roughly chopped into ½-inch pieces

¼ cup extra-virgin olive oil

½ teaspoon Calabrian chile paste

½ teaspoon kosher salt

FOR THE FISH

Vegetable oil cooking spray

4 skinless center-cut salmon fillets (about 5 ounces each)

¾ teaspoon kosher salt

1 teaspoon grated lemon zest

1 teaspoon olive oil

Lemon wedges, for serving

Place an oven rack in the top third of the oven and preheat the broiler. Spray a rimmed baking sheet with cooking spray.

Place the potato in a large saucepan, add water to cover by 3 inches, and season generously with salt. Bring to a boil over medium-high heat and cook until the potato chunks are tender when pierced with a fork, about 5 minutes. Add the chopped broccoli and boil for another 4 to 5 minutes, until the stems are tender.

Drain the vegetables and transfer to a large bowl. Add the extra-virgin olive oil, chile paste, and ½ teaspoon salt. Using a potato masher or a whisk, crush the mixture until it resembles rustic mashed potatoes. Cover to keep warm while you broil the salmon.

Arrange the salmon fillets on the prepared baking sheet and sprinkle evenly with the salt and lemon zest. Rub the fillets with the olive oil. Broil for 6 to 8 minutes, until just cooked through and slightly golden brown. To serve, spoon some of the broccoli mash onto each plate and top with a salmon fillet. Serve with lemon wedges on the side.

ROASTED TROUT WITH HAZELNUT GREMOLATA

SERVES 2

Freshwater fish like trout is less likely to harbor heavy metals than big ocean fish, and I love its mild, clean flavor. Ask your fishmonger to fillet them for you or simply stuff them and roast them whole.

FOR THE GREMOLATA

¼ cup skinless toasted hazelnuts (see Note)

½ cup chopped fresh flat-leaf parsley

¼ cup olive oil

1 teaspoon grated lemon zest

1 tablespoon fresh lemon juice, from ½ lemon

½ teaspoon kosher salt

FOR THE FISH

1 (8-ounce) package cremini mushrooms, sliced ⅓ inch thick

1 small acorn squash, halved lengthwise, seeds removed, and sliced crosswise into ¼-inch half-moons

1 teaspoons kosher salt

1 tablespoon plus 2 teaspoons olive oil

2 rainbow trout, filleted (4 small fillets)

Position one oven rack in the top third of the oven and another in the bottom third. Preheat the oven to 450°F.

In a small bowl, combine the hazelnuts, parsley, olive oil, lemon zest, lemon juice, and ½ teaspoon salt. Mix well to combine.

In a medium bowl, toss together the mushrooms, squash, ½ teaspoon of the salt, and 1 tablespoon of the olive oil. Spread the mixture on a rimmed baking sheet and roast in the bottom third of the oven for 12 minutes, or until the squash is tender and beginning to brown. Remove the vegetables from the oven and preheat the broiler to high.

Using a sharp knife, make three diagonal slashes on the skin side of each fillet. Season the fillets evenly with the remaining ½ teaspoon salt and rub each one with ½ teaspoon of the oil.

Place the fillets, skin side up, on the top rack in the oven, above the roasted vegetables. Broil for 8 to 9 minutes, or until the skin is lightly browned and crisp and the flesh is cooked through but still moist.

Place some of the vegetables on each serving plate and top with the fish. Spoon the gremolata over the fish.

NOTE ————

Toast hazelnuts in a 350°F oven for 5 minutes, or until lightly browned. While still warm, rub the nuts between your hands to remove most of the skins.

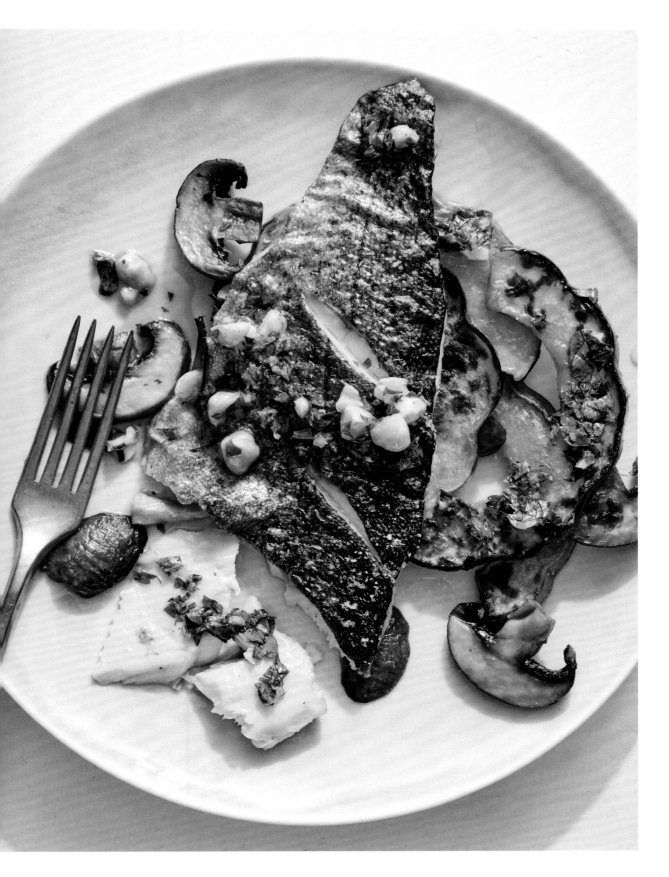

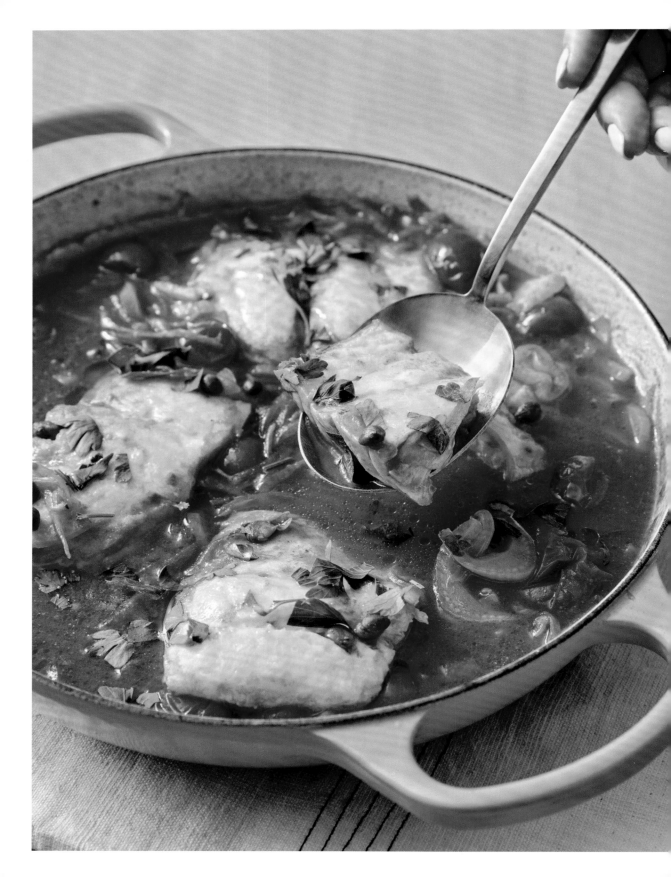

AQUA PAZZA

SERVES 4

Aqua pazza was one of my grandfather Dino's favorite dishes, especially for a Sunday afternoon lunch. The name means "crazy water," a reference to the way the wine and oil in the cooking liquid stay separate in the bowl, making the sauce look broken—or maybe the name just means it's crazy good! I usually make this with big, beautiful chunks of sea bass, but it would work with any meaty fish, including monkfish, salmon, cod, or even scallops. Traditionally it's served on its own like a hearty fish stew, with a big hunk of bread, but it would also be great ladled over lentils, brown rice, or greens.

2 tablespoons olive oil

2 garlic cloves, smashed and peeled

1 red onion, halved and thinly sliced

1 fennel bulb, stalks removed, halved and thinly sliced

½ teaspoon crushed red pepper flakes

1 teaspoon kosher salt

½ cup white wine

1 (14-ounce) can cherry tomatoes

2 tablespoons drained capers

4 skinless red snapper or striped bass fillets (6 ounces each)

2 tablespoons chopped fresh flat-leaf parsley

Extra-virgin olive oil, to finish

Heat a 12-inch straight-sided skillet or shallow braiser over medium-high heat. Add the olive oil, garlic, onion, fennel, and red pepper flakes. Season with ½ teaspoon of the salt. Cook, stirring often with a wooden spoon, for about 5 minutes, or until the vegetables are soft and fragrant. Add the wine and stir, scraping up any bits from the bottom of the pan. Add the tomatoes, capers, and 1 cup water and bring to a simmer. Reduce the heat to medium-low to maintain a gentle simmer and cook for 10 minutes.

Season the fillets with the remaining ½ teaspoon salt. Slide the fillets into the broth and cover the pan with a tight-fitting lid. Cook for 12 to 15 minutes, until the fish is firm and opaque all the way through. Remove the lid and spoon some of the sauce over the fish. Sprinkle with parsley, drizzle with a bit of extra-virgin olive oil, and serve.

SHEET PAN PARMESAN SHRIMP *and* VEGGIES

SERVES 4

Back in the day, one-pan dinners used to mean a heavy casserole, a far cry from this beautiful, fresh, easy-peasy crowd-pleaser. Just let the veggies caramelize a bit, add the shrimp, and cook for another 10 minutes, until everything is nice and crispy—bang, dinner is ready! Serve it over arugula or with a salad to make sure you get your greens in too.

1 small broccoli crown, cut into 1-inch florets

1 red onion, cut into 1-inch dice

½ medium cauliflower, cut into 1-inch florets

1 cup grape or cherry tomatoes

4 tablespoons olive oil

1½ teaspoons kosher salt

1 pound large shrimp, peeled and deveined

½ cup freshly grated Parmigiano-Reggiano

½ teaspoon dried oregano

2 tablespoons gluten-free or regular panko (optional)

1 lemon

Preheat the oven to 450°F.

In a large bowl, mix the broccoli, onion, cauliflower, tomatoes, 3 tablespoons of the olive oil, and 1 teaspoon of the salt. Spread the vegetables on a rimmed baking sheet and roast for about 15 minutes, until cooked through and just beginning to brown.

Meanwhile, combine the shrimp, Parmigiano, oregano, the remaining 1 tablespoon oil, and the remaining ½ teaspoon salt to the same bowl that was used for the vegetables. Toss well to coat evenly in the cheese and oregano. Remove the vegetables from the oven and scatter the shrimp on top. Stir gently to combine and sprinkle with the panko, if using.

Return to the oven for 8 to 10 minutes, until the shrimp are pink and cooked through. Grate the zest from the lemon over the mixture and toss to combine. Cut the zested lemon into wedges and serve with the shrimp and veggies.

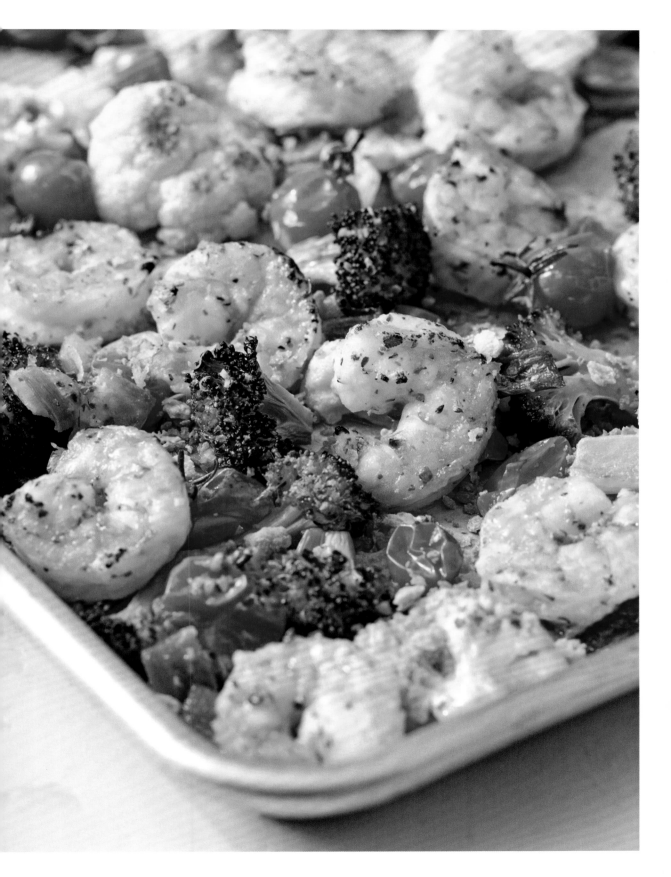

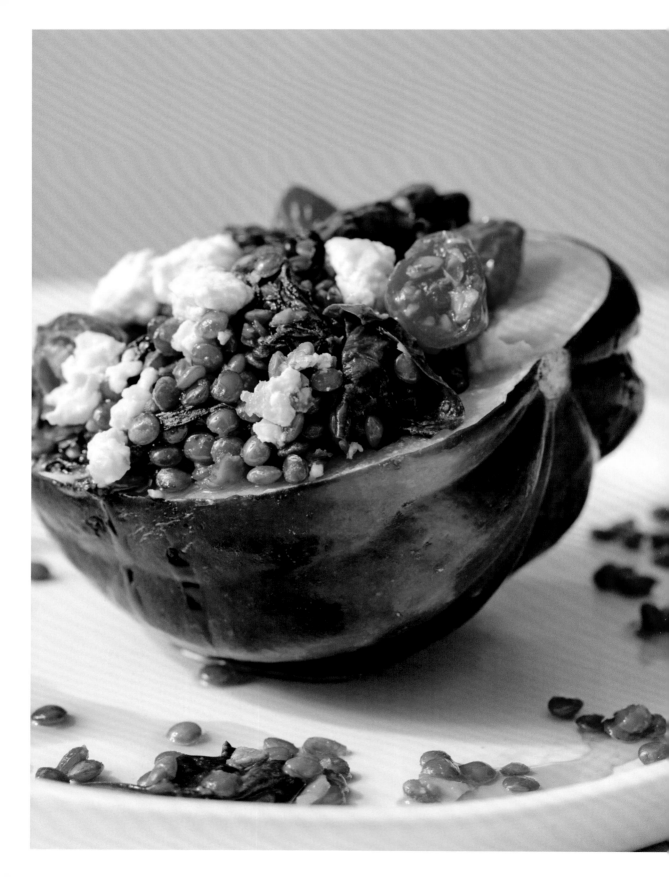

LENTIL-STUFFED SQUASH

My mom became a vegetarian when I was a teenager, and stuffed vegetable entrées like this one were on the table a *lot*. She especially liked lentils and stuffed them into everything from bell peppers to hollowed-out onions. I've taken that idea and applied it to a very American vegetable: acorn squash. It's a dish that's got everything I need for a meal, and it's is also just really delicious looking!

2 tablespoons olive oil

1 shallot, chopped

1 garlic clove, chopped

1½ teaspoons kosher salt

1 cup green lentils, rinsed

2 fresh oregano sprigs

½ cup chopped cherry tomatoes

2½ cups (packed) chopped baby spinach

¼ cup (packed) chopped basil leaves

½ cup crumbled feta or goat cheese

2 medium acorn or delicata squash, halved lengthwise and seeded

Preheat the oven to 400°F.

Heat a saucepan over medium heat. Add the oil, shallot, garlic, and ½ teaspoon of the salt and cook, stirring often, for about 3 minutes, or until the shallot is soft and fragrant. Add the lentils and stir to coat in all the flavors. Add the oregano sprigs and 1½ cups water and bring to a simmer. Reduce the heat to low, cover, and simmer for 20 minutes, or until the lentils are just cooked through.

Discard the oregano sprigs and add the tomatoes, spinach, basil, ½ teaspoon of the salt, and ¼ cup of the feta to the lentils. Stir until the spinach is completely wilted and the tomatoes are warmed through.

Arrange the squash halves cut side up in a baking dish. Season the squash with the remaining ½ teaspoon salt. Divide the lentil mixture among the squash halves. Dot with the remaining ¼ cup cheese.

Pour 1 cup water into the baking dish and cover it loosely with aluminum foil. Bake the squash for 30 minutes, or until tender when pierced with the tip of a knife. Serve warm.

BEYOND STUFFED PEPPERS

SERVES 4

I've been trying to add more recipes incorporating meat alternatives into my repertoire, and this was one of the first things I tried. Bell peppers are a great vehicle for just about any kind of stuffing, and the peppers themselves are so flavorful and colorful that the dish feels and tastes familiar even without the usual lamb or beef filling. I make this often when I have guests who don't eat meat, as it makes a lovely presentation.

4 medium red, yellow, or orange bell peppers

½ teaspoons kosher salt

2 tablespoons olive oil

½ pound plant-based "ground meat," such as Beyond Meat, thawed if frozen

2 shallots, chopped

1 fennel bulb, stalks removed, chopped into ⅓-inch pieces

¼ teaspoon dried oregano

1½ cups cooked brown rice (page 94)

1 (14-ounce) can cherry tomatoes, crushed by hand

¼ cup fresh basil, chopped

1 cup baby spinach, chopped

½ cup freshly grated Parmigiano-Reggiano

¾ cup grated Provolone or mozzarella cheese

Preheat the oven to 375°F.

Cut off the top ⅓ inch of each pepper and pull out the ribs and seeds. Chop the caps into ⅓-inch pieces, discarding the stems. Cut a thin slice off the bottom from each pepper so that they stand upright. Season the insides evenly with ¼ teaspoon of the salt. Nestle the peppers in a baking dish that holds them snuggly and set aside.

Heat a large skillet over medium-high heat. Add the oil and heat for another minute, then add the "ground meat" and use the back of a wooden spoon to break it into small pieces. Cook, stirring occasionally, until the crumbles are browned, about 5 minutes. Add the chopped pepper caps, shallots, fennel, oregano, and the remaining 1¼ teaspoons salt and cook another 4 minutes, or until fragrant and the vegetables are beginning to soften. Stir in the rice, tomatoes, basil, spinach, and Parmigiano cheese and continue to cook until the spinach is wilted and the cheese is melted, about 3 minutes.

Spoon the mixture into the peppers, dividing it evenly, and top with the Provolone. Add ½ cup water to the baking dish. Bake the peppers for 40 minutes, or until the cheese is melted and the peppers are soft but not collapsing. Serve hot.

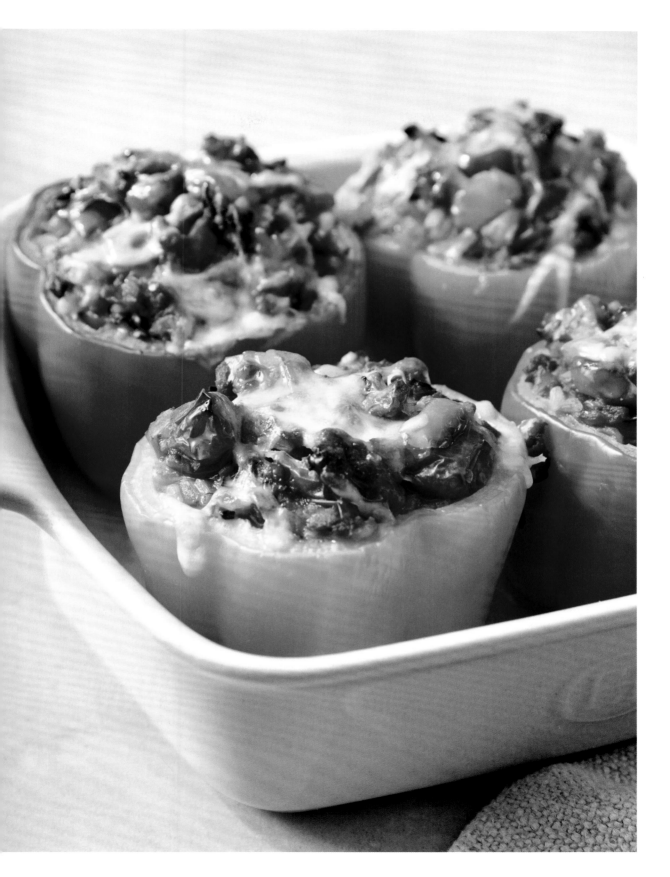

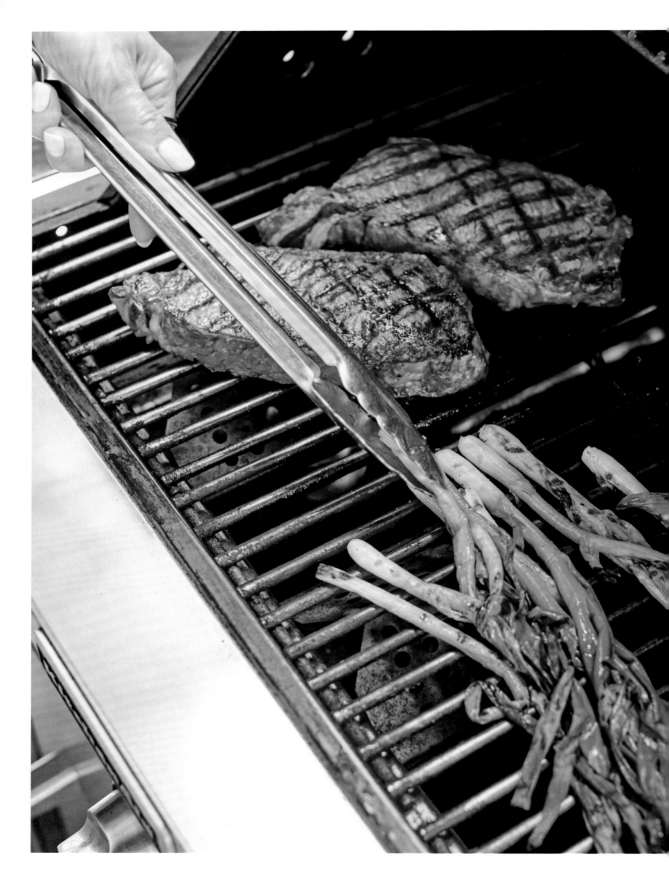

GRILLED STRIP STEAK WITH SCALLION SALSA VERDE

SERVES 4

If you're a steakhouse person, or cook for one on the regular, this grilled strip steak should definitely be in your playbook. Make a double batch of the green sauce, because once you've tried it, you will want to put it on *everything*. I serve it with lamb chops, chicken, any kind of seafood—it even works as a chunky salad dressing. It should go without saying that you can also cook the steak on either a gas or charcoal grill.

2 (1½-inch) New York strip steaks (about 1¾ pounds total)

1½ teaspoons kosher salt

FOR THE SAUCE

2 bunches of scallions or ramps

¾ teaspoon kosher salt

2 tablespoons plus 1 teaspoon olive oil

2 teaspoons whole-grain mustard

2 teaspoons cider vinegar

Preheat the oven to 400°F. Remove the steaks from the refrigerator 15 minutes before cooking.

Heat a ridged grill pan over medium-high heat. Dry the steaks well with paper towels and season them evenly with 1½ teaspoons salt. Place the steaks on the hot grill pan. Cook for 5 minutes per side, or until deep golden brown on the bottom. Without turning off the heat under the grill pan, transfer the steaks to a rimmed baking sheet and place in the oven for about 5 minutes for medium, or until an instant-read thermometer inserted in the center of a steak registers 135°F. Transfer to a rack to rest for 10 minutes.

Meanwhile, make the sauce: Season the scallions with ¼ teaspoon of the salt and 1 teaspoon of the olive oil. Place on the hot grill pan and grill for about 3 minutes per side, or until wilted and slightly charred. Coarsely chop the scallions, then place them in a small bowl along with the mustard, vinegar, and the remaining 2 tablespoons olive oil and ½ teaspoon salt. Stir to combine.

Slice the steaks across the grain and serve with the scallion sauce spooned on top.

PAN-ROASTED PORK CHOPS WITH CHERRY *and* RED WINE SAUCE

SERVES 4

Not all pork is created equal: if you can find a good heritage breed, like Berkshire, the difference in taste is really notable and worth an occasional splurge. Because it is so flavorful, I find one big beautiful chop, nicely carved off the bone, will feed two people. The cherry and wine sauce really brings out the sweetness of the pork; just make sure to buy cherries with no added sugar, because they are plenty sweet all on their own.

2 thick bone-in pork loin chops (10 to 12 ounces each)

3 tablespoons olive oil

1½ teaspoons kosher salt

1 shallot, chopped

1 cup halved frozen cherries, slightly thawed

1 cup dry, fruity, light red wine, such as Pinot Noir

1 tablespoon Dijon mustard

Preheat the oven to 400°F. Remove the pork chops from the refrigerator 10 minutes before cooking.

Heat a large skillet over medium-high heat. Add 2 tablespoons of the olive oil and heat for another minute. Dry the pork well with paper towels and season with 1 teaspoon of the salt. Place the chops in the pan and cook without moving them for 4 minutes, or until they are deep golden brown on the bottom. Flip the chops and cook for an additional 4 minutes to brown the second side. Transfer the chops to a rimmed baking sheet and cook in the oven for 5 minutes, or until an instant-read thermometer inserted in the thickest part registers 140°F. Allow to rest for 10 minutes before serving.

While the chops are in the oven, put the shallot and the remaining ½ teaspoon salt in the pan that the pork was seared in. Cook over medium-high heat for 1 minute, stirring often with a wooden spoon. Reduce the heat to medium and stir in the cherries and the wine, scraping the bottom of the pan to loosen the browned bits. Whisk in the mustard. Stir in the remaining 1 tablespoon olive oil and increase the heat to bring the sauce to a boil. Boil for 5 to 10 minutes to emulsify and reduce it by a third. Spoon the sauce over the pork and serve.

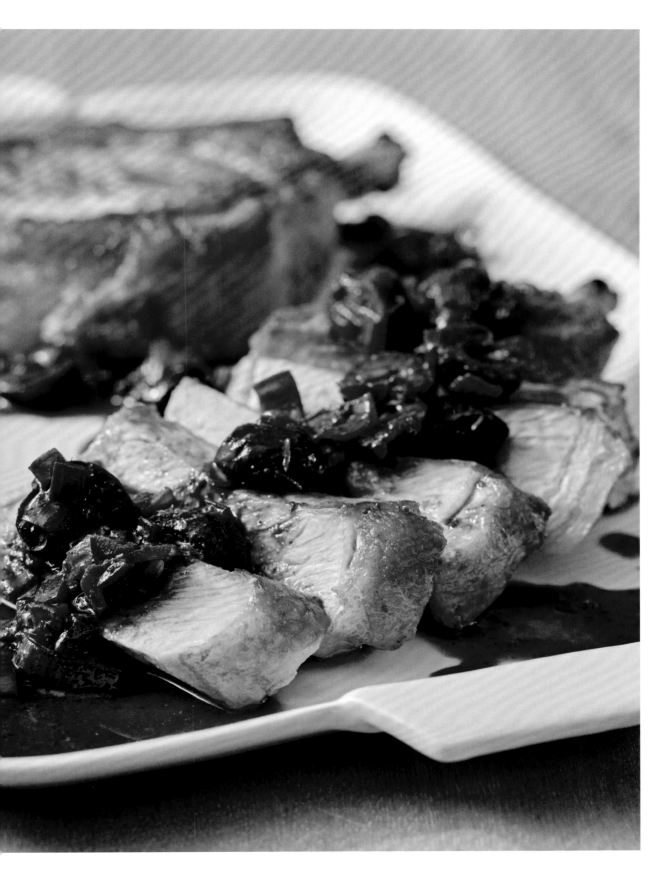

TENDERLOIN FILETS WITH SWEET OLIVE TAPENADE

SERVES 4

I don't eat beef more than once or twice a month, so when I do, I like it to be a little special. Beef tenderloin, aka filet mignon, is one of the leanest cuts, so I like to pair it with something rich but not necessarily creamy, like this deca-dent topping made with buttery green olives brightened with citrus. Slice the tenderloins and serve them over a bed of greens for a superfast company meal.

FOR THE TAPENADE

½ cup olive oil

2 shallots, chopped into ⅓-inch pieces

1 cup pitted green olives, such as Castelvetrano or Cerignola

1 teaspoon grated lemon zest

1 teaspoon fresh lemon juice

2 teaspoons chopped fresh oregano

FOR THE STEAK

2 tablespoons olive oil

4 center-cut beef filets (about 6 ounces each)

2 teaspoons kosher salt

½ lemon

Combine the olive oil and shallots in a small saucepan. Place over medium-low heat and cook gently for 15 minutes, or until the shallots are tender all the way through but not browned. Remove from the heat to cool slightly.

Combine the olives, lemon zest, lemon juice, and oregano in a food processor and pulse a few times to combine. Use a slotted spoon to transfer the shallots to the food processor. Add ¼ cup of the oil from the shallots and pulse until combined but still slightly chunky. (Save the extra shallot oil for a salad dressing or another use.) Set aside to allow the flavors to marry.

Preheat the oven to 400°F.

Heat an ovenproof skillet over medium-high heat. Add the oil to the pan and heat for an additional minute. Dry the steaks well with paper towels and season with the salt. Place the steaks in the pan and cook without moving them for 3 minutes, or until a deep golden crust forms on the bottom.

Flip the steaks and cook for an additional 3 minutes, then carefully transfer the skillet to the oven. Roast the steaks for 5 minutes, or until an instant-read thermometer inserted in the side registers 135°F for medium. Transfer the steaks to a plate and squeeze the lemon half over them. Let the steaks rest for 10 minutes before serving, topped with the tapenade.

LAMB *and* RED WINE STEW

SERVES 4

Lamb is my go-to red meat, and I tend to eat it more often than beef, especially in braised dishes like this one, where it creates such a flavorful pan sauce. Served with roasted potatoes or a baked sweet potato to sop up the juices, it is deeply satisfying, and even better the day after it's made. This isn't weeknight fare for me, and not only because it takes some time to cook; it's the kind of rich, rib-sticking dish I enjoy most when it's the exception, not the rule, so I save it for a winter weekend.

2 tablespoons olive oil

1 pound lamb stew meat, cut into 1-inch cubes

2 teaspoons kosher salt

3 carrots, diced

1 onion, diced

2 celery stalks, diced

2 garlic cloves, smashed and peeled

2 tablespoons rice flour

2 tablespoons tomato paste

1½ cups dry red wine

1½ cups low-sodium beef broth

1 bay leaf

5 fresh thyme sprigs

1 cup green Cerignola olives, smashed and pitted

2 tablespoons chopped fresh flat-leaf parsley

Place a medium Dutch oven over medium-high heat. Add the olive oil and heat for 30 seconds. Dry the lamb cubes well with paper towels and season with 1½ teaspoons of the salt. Place the lamb in the hot pan and cook without moving it for 4 minutes, or until deeply browned on one side. Using tongs to flip the meat, continue to brown the lamb pieces for about 4 minutes per side, until evenly browned on all sides, about 20 minutes total. Transfer to a plate.

Add the carrots, onion, celery, and garlic to the pan. Season with the remaining ½ teaspoon salt and cook, stirring often, for about 5 minutes, or until the vegetables are fragrant and beginning to soften. Stir in the flour and tomato paste and cook for another minute. Add the wine and use a wooden spoon to loosen the browned bits from the bottom of the pan. Bring to a simmer and cook for 5 minutes to reduce slightly, stirring often. Stir in the broth, bay leaf, thyme, and browned meat and reduce the heat to medium-low to maintain a gentle simmer. Cover and simmer for 1 hour.

After 1 hour, stir in the olives. Cover the pan, leaving the lid slightly askew to allow steam to escape, and simmer for an additional 30 minutes, or until the meat is completely tender. Discard the bay leaf. Stir in the parsley and serve.

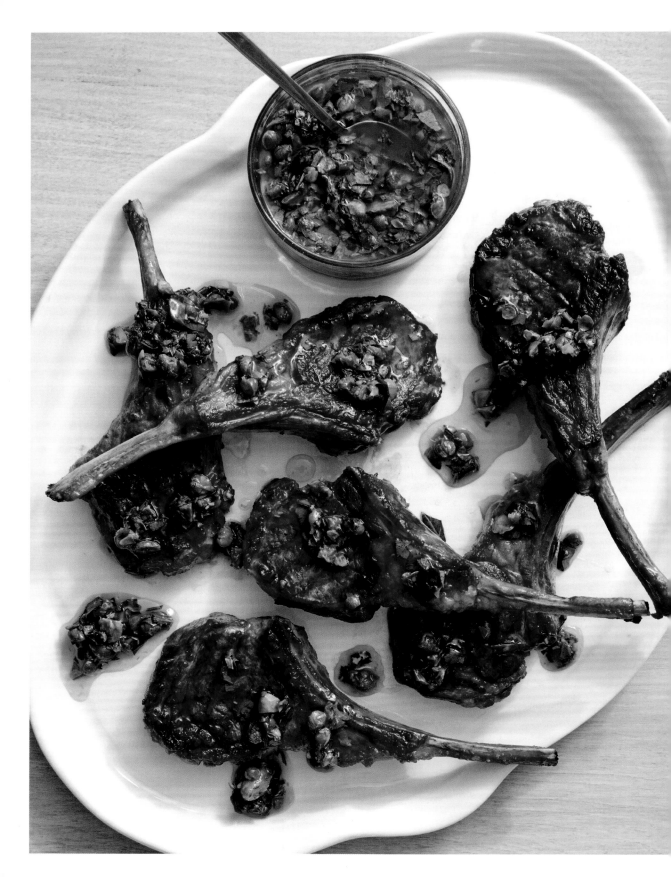

LAMB CHOPS
WITH MINT *and* PISTACHIO SALSA VERDE

SERVES 6

I have noticed that even people who don't think they love lamb enjoy tender rib chops because they are just fun to eat; when you french the chops (scraping off the fat and meat to expose the long rib bones—most butchers can do this for you), they are like little lollipops you can hold in your fingers. If you serve the lamb over quinoa or another grain, the salsa verde will bring all the elements together into a filling entrée, even though it's a relatively modest serving of meat.

FOR THE SALSA VERDE

½ cup chopped fresh
   flat-leaf parsley

¼ cup chopped fresh mint

2 tablespoons drained
   capers, chopped

¼ cup chopped roasted,
   lightly salted pistachios

½ cup olive oil

1 tablespoon fresh lemon
   juice, from ½ lemon

½ teaspoon kosher salt

FOR THE LAMB

12 frenched rib lamb chops

1¼ teaspoons kosher salt

Olive oil, for the pan

In a medium bowl, combine the parsley, mint, capers, pistachios, olive oil, and lemon juice. Season with ½ teaspoon salt and stir with a rubber spatula to combine. Set aside to let the flavors marry while you cook the meat.

Meanwhile, heat a ridged grill pan over medium-high heat. Dry the lamb chops well with paper towels and season with 1¼ teaspoons salt. Brush the pan with olive oil and cook the chops for 4 minutes on each side for medium rare. Transfer to a plate to rest for 10 minutes.

Serve the chops drizzled with some of the salsa verde and pass the remaining sauce at the table.

CHAPTER 14

The Side Hustle

Since opening my restaurants, I've become much more aware of the way a great side dish can sell a meal. Roast chicken with rice and green beans? Sure, fine. Roast chicken with Cauliflower–Sweet Potato Mash and Green Bean "Fries"? Yes, please!! All of the recipes in this section turn even simple entrées into *yes, please* moments, and many of them are special enough to anchor a meal, either all on their own or supplemented by some of the ready-to-go components from the batch chapter (page 78) that you've been cooking up and stashing in the fridge. However you choose to serve them, each one of these sides is a meal-maker.

And don't forget to draw down from your store of big-batch recipes when you want a nearly instant side; those go-with-anything greens and grains are lifesavers when you need dinner on the table yesterday!

SIMPLE SALAD OF BITTER GREENS

SERVES 4 TO 6

Chicories, like radicchio, endive, and Treviso, are no shrinking violets; their mildly bitter edge makes them assertive enough to stand up to even boldly flavored entrées. The lemony dressing adds brightness to any heavy meal. You can prep the leaves ahead of time, but don't dress them until you're ready to serve or the arugula will become limp and soggy.

1 head of radicchio, cut into 1-inch pieces

1 large or 2 small Belgian endives, cut into ½-inch pieces

1 head of Treviso or baby frisée, cut into ½-inch pieces

2 cups baby arugula

1½ tablespoons fresh lemon juice, from 1 lemon

2 tablespoons extra-virgin olive oil

1 teaspoon kosher salt

In a large bowl, combine the radicchio, endive, Treviso, arugula, lemon juice, olive oil, and salt. Use your hands to toss the greens gently and coat them evenly with the dressing.

CREAMY DILL COLESLAW

SERVES 6 TO 8

I get the appeal of traditional coleslaw's crunchy texture and fresh flavor, but I've never really warmed up to heavy mayonnaise dressings. Coconut yogurt gives this picnic staple the same creaminess, but it's a lot lighter. I especially like how the seeds in whole-grain mustard provide little pops of extra flavor. Massaging the cabbage with a bit of salt infuses it with flavor and also tenderizes it, so don't skip that step!

1 medium head of savoy cabbage, quartered, core removed, and sliced fine

1 tablespoon plus 1 teaspoon kosher salt

¾ cup coconut yogurt, such as COYO

1 tablespoon whole-grain mustard

3 tablespoons cider vinegar

¼ cup extra-virgin olive oil

¼ cup chopped fresh dill

1 carrot, grated on the large holes of a box grater

In a large colander, toss the cabbage with 1 tablespoon kosher salt. With your hands, massage the salt into the cabbage for about 3 minutes. Place the colander in the sink and let the cabbage drain for 15 minutes.

Meanwhile, in a large bowl, whisk together the yogurt, mustard, vinegar, olive oil, dill, and the remaining 1 teaspoon salt until smooth. Add the carrot and stir to coat. Squeeze out any excess liquid from the cabbage and add the cabbage to the bowl, tossing well to combine with the carrots and dressing. Let the slaw stand at room temperature for 30 minutes or up to 4 hours in the refrigerator to marry the flavors.

MISTA SALAD WITH ROASTED GARLIC DRESSING

SERVES 4 TO 6

People are always surprised when I tell them the "secret" ingredient in this salad is a whole head of roasted garlic in the dressing. It makes a thick, slightly sweet puree with none of the sharpness of raw garlic, and it clings to the salad greens beautifully. Topped with shards of nutty Parmigiano-Reggiano and crispy capers, it's a very special dish, perfect when you want to bring something to a friend's house that's a notch above a plain green salad.

FOR THE ROASTED GARLIC

1 head of garlic, unpeeled

2 tablespoons olive oil

¼ teaspoon kosher salt

FOR THE FRIED CAPERS

About ½ cup olive oil

3 tablespoons drained capers

FOR THE DRESSING

¼ cup roasted garlic

2 teaspoons Dijon mustard

2 tablespoons fresh lemon
  juice, from 1 lemon

2 tablespoons olive oil

¼ teaspoon kosher salt

FOR THE SALAD

2 small heads of Treviso or 1
  small radicchio, sliced

1 fennel bulb, stalks removed,
  very thinly sliced crosswise

1 cup cherry tomatoes, halved

¼ teaspoon kosher salt

3 ounces Parmigiano-
  Reggiano, shaved

Preheat the oven to 350°F.

Roast the garlic: Cut the top third off the head of garlic and discard or save it for another use. Place the remaining head in the center of a piece of aluminum foil large enough to enclose it completely. Drizzle it with olive oil, sprinkle with salt, and bring the foil up around the top, sealing it well. Roast for 45 minutes, or until the garlic is lightly browned and very soft. Allow to cool slightly.

While the garlic roasts, fry the capers: Pour ½ cup olive oil into a small saucepan—the oil should be about ½ inch deep—and heat over medium heat. When hot, add the capers and fry until opened, golden brown, and crispy, 2 to 3 minutes. Transfer to a paper-towel-lined plate to drain.

To make the dressing, squeeze the cooled head of garlic from the bottom to remove all the cloves. Measure ¼ cup of the garlic (save any extra for another use) and place in a small blender or food processor. Add the mustard, lemon juice, olive oil, and salt. Puree on medium-high speed until emulsified and smooth.

Place the Treviso, fennel, and cherry tomatoes in a large bowl and sprinkle with the salt. Drizzle with the dressing and toss well to coat. Sprinkle with the cheese shavings and the crispy capers and serve.

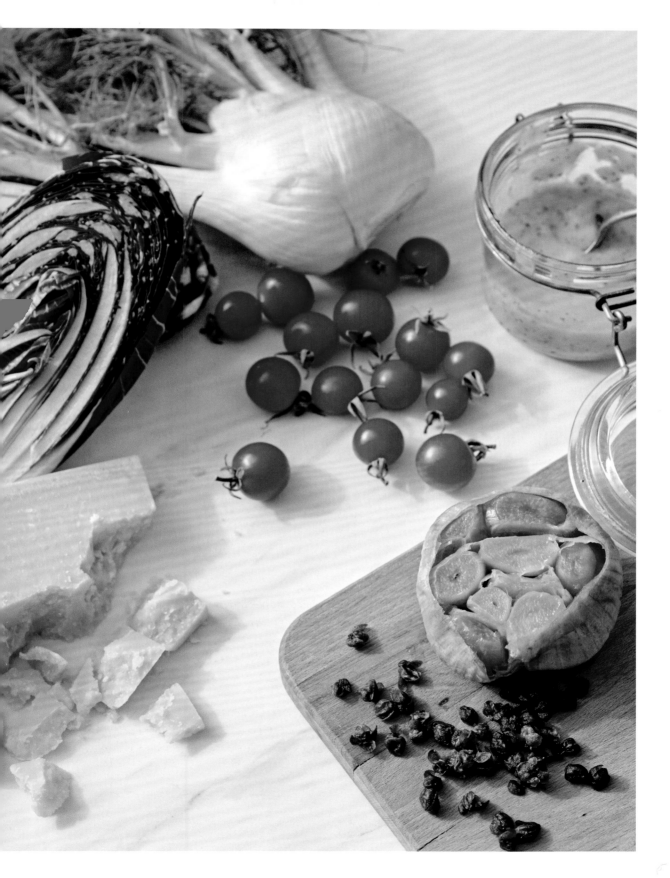

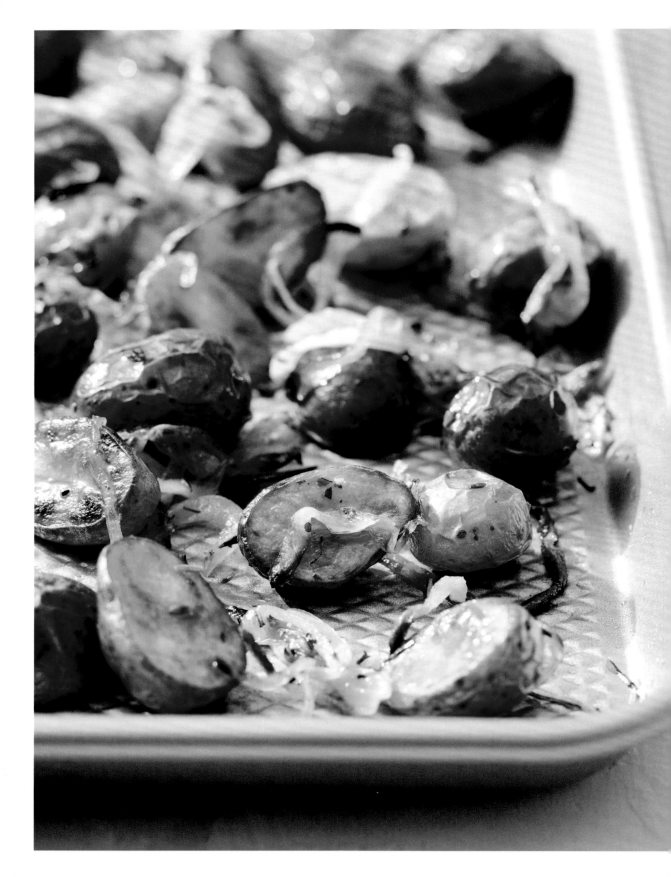

HERBES DE PROVENCE
ROASTED POTATOES

SERVES 4 TO 6

I've been making this forever, and I never get tired of it. Don't leave out the onion; its caramelized sweetness is what makes the dish. I love to use marble-size Peewee potatoes, which are about an inch in diameter; you could use halved baby Yukon Golds, red new potatoes, or a mixture instead.

24 ounces golden Peewee potatoes, whole or other small potatoes, halved

1 medium onion, halved and sliced

⅓ cup olive oil

1 tablespoon herbes de Provence

1 teaspoon kosher salt

Position a rack in the lower third of the oven. Preheat the oven to 450°F.

Mound the potatoes and onion on a rimmed baking sheet and drizzle with the oil. Sprinkle with the dried herbs and salt and toss well to coat evenly. Spread out the potatoes on the baking sheet and roast them on the lower rack for 30 to 35 minutes, until golden brown and tender. Serve warm.

(RB)

CRISPY ROASTED
BROCCOLI

SERVES 4

You can jazz up this simple side any way you and your family like by season-ing the broccoli right on the baking sheet just before you serve it. If you like things spicy, toss the broccoli with ¼ teaspoon or more of crushed red pepper flakes; for a brighter flavor, grate some lemon zest onto the florets and give them a toss. And a light dusting of Parm will get Jade to eat almost anything.

2 broccoli crowns, cut into 1-inch florets

3 tablespoons olive oil

1 teaspoon kosher salt

Optional seasonings: ¼ teaspoon crushed red pepper flakes, grated zest of ½ lemon, or 3 tablespoons grated Parmigiano-Reggiano

Position a rack in the lower third of the oven. Preheat the oven to 450°F.

On a rimmed baking sheet, toss together the broccoli, olive oil, and salt. Spread the broccoli evenly on the baking sheet and roast on the lower rack for 25 minutes, flipping the pieces halfway through. Sprinkle with one or more of the optional seasonings, if desired, and serve warm.

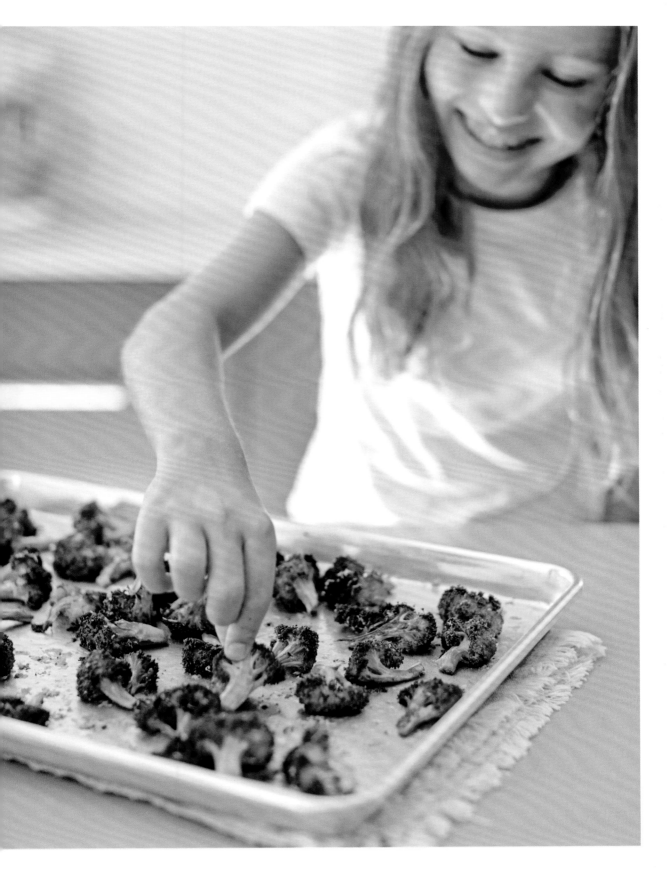

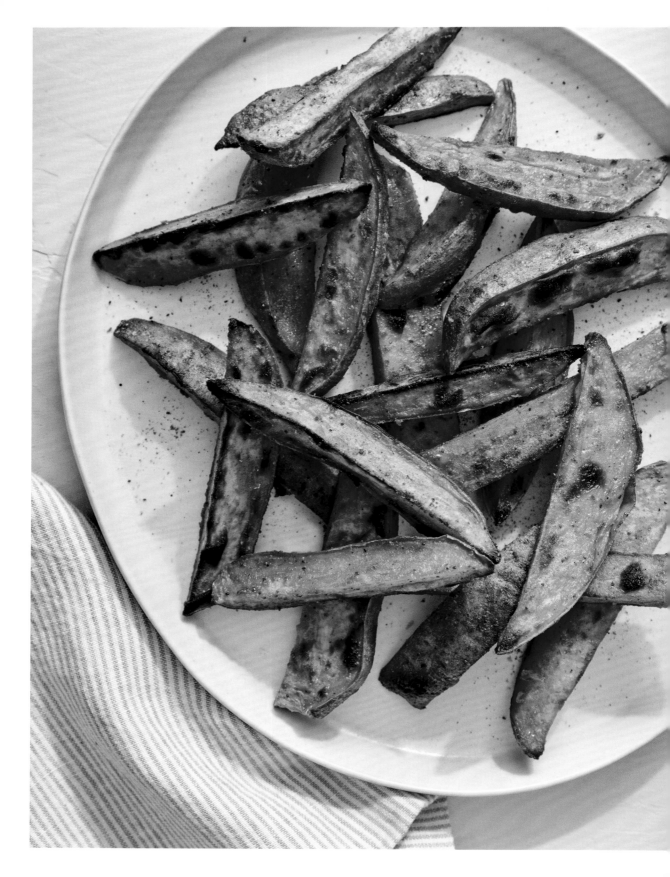

GIGI'S SWEET POTATO WEDGES

SERVES 4

Gigi cooked for my grandfather Dino and has been part of my family for nearly forty years. Dino was crazy for these potatoes and all of his grandchildren, me included, gobbled them up too.

3 small sweet potatoes, scrubbed but not peeled, cut into 1-inch wedges

2 tablespoons olive oil

1½ tablespoons Old Bay seasoning

Preheat the oven to 450°F. Place a rimmed baking sheet in the oven as it preheats.

In a medium bowl, toss together the sweet potatoes, olive oil, and Old Bay. Using an oven mitt, remove the hot baking sheet from the oven and pour the wedges onto the tray, spreading them in a single layer. Roast for 25 minutes, or until deep golden brown and beginning to crisp, flipping the wedges halfway through.

GREEN BEAN "FRIES"

Although these aren't really fried, like french fries, they are fun finger food that goes great with a burger or grilled dish. Prepared this way, the beans are similar to grilled shishito peppers in taste and texture, but without the spicy bite, making them a little more kid-friendly. They take a few minutes to blister, but be patient—those dark, almost charred spots are what gives them so much flavor. Serve with your favorite dip or simply with a squeeze of lemon.

2 tablespoons olive oil

½ pound green beans, trimmed

¼ teaspoon kosher salt

Heat a large skillet over medium-high heat for 3 minutes. Carefully add the oil and heat for another minute. Scatter the beans evenly in the pan and season with the salt. (If the pan is too small to allow all the beans to make contact with the bottom of the pan, cook them in two batches.) Cook the beans without moving them for 3 minutes, or until browned, blistered, and beginning to split on the bottom.

Using tongs or a slotted spatula, flip the beans and cook for another 2 minutes. Flip one more time and cook for another minute, or until all the beans have a good amount of golden brown patches. Drain on a paper-towel-lined plate. Serve hot.

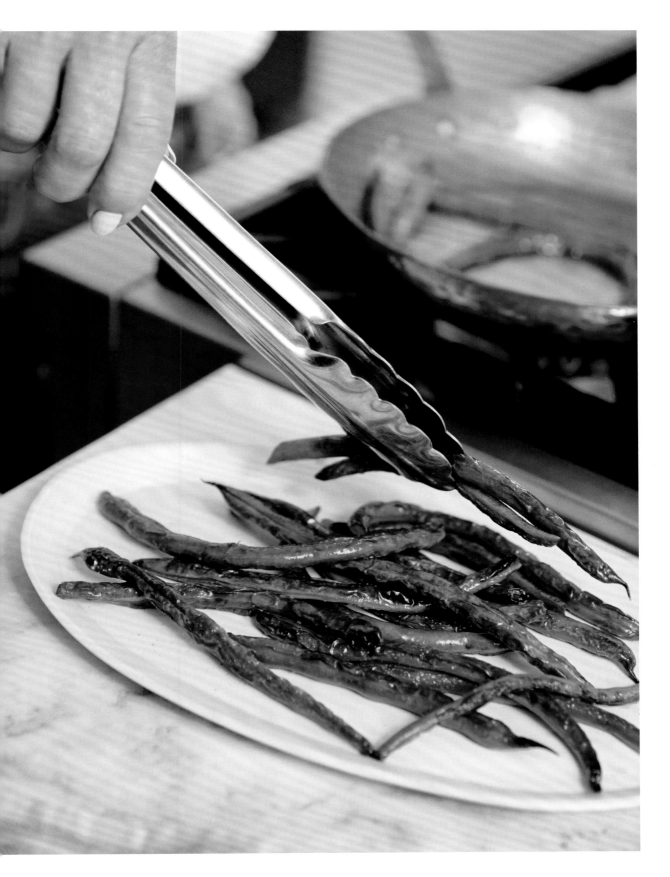

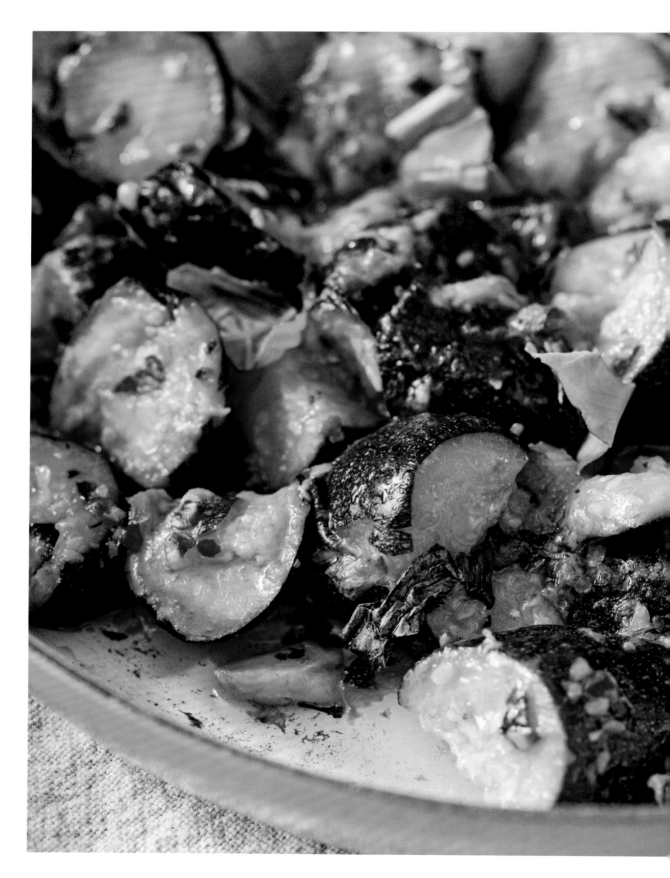

BRAISED ZUCCHINI WITH BASIL

When zucchini is cooked this way, it creates an interesting mix of textures. Some pieces get soft and almost creamy, while others retain a little crunch. It's bright and satisfying, all in one zippy bite.

3 tablespoons olive oil

2 garlic cloves, smashed and peeled

½ teaspoon crushed red pepper flakes

4 medium zucchini (about 2 pounds total), cut into 1-inch pieces

1¼ teaspoons kosher salt

½ cup vegetable or chicken broth, homemade (page 95 or 96) or low-sodium store-bought

¼ cup chopped fresh basil

1 teaspoon grated lemon zest

1 teaspoon fresh lemon juice

Heat a large Dutch oven over medium-high heat. Add 2 tablespoons of the oil and heat for an additional 30 seconds. Add the garlic and cook until light golden brown and fragrant, about 2 minutes. Add the red pepper flakes, zucchini, and salt to the pan and cook, stirring often, for about 6 minutes, or until the zucchini is starting to soften and brown in spots. Add the broth and cover.

Reduce the heat to low and cook for 5 minutes. Remove the cover, raise the heat to medium-high, and cook for an additional 5 minutes to reduce the liquid by half. Some zucchini will be quite soft and some will retain a slight bite. Stir in the remaining tablespoon of oil and the basil, lemon zest, and lemon juice and serve.

SIMPLE BRAISED MUSHROOMS

SERVES 6

This is one very versatile side dish, and it has less fat than most sautéed mushrooms, with just 1 tablespoon of butter stirred in at the end for flavor. The mushrooms can be served as is, but leftovers are great in a frittata or risotto, or spooned over chicken as a sauce. They are simple and sophisticated and screaming with mushroom flavor.

2 tablespoons olive oil

1 shallot, finely chopped

1½ teaspoons kosher salt

3 (10-ounce) packages cremini mushrooms, trimmed and quartered

4 fresh thyme sprigs

2 tablespoons dry Marsala, sherry, or white wine (optional)

½ cup chicken or vegetable broth, homemade (page 96 or 95) or low-sodium store-bought

1 tablespoon unsalted butter

Heat a large straight-sided skillet over medium-high heat. Add the oil and heat for 30 seconds. Add the shallot and ½ teaspoon of the salt and cook, stirring often, for 2 minutes, or until fragrant and beginning to soften. Add the mushrooms to the pan along with another ½ teaspoon of the salt and the thyme. Cook, stirring often, until the mushrooms have released some of their juices and are beginning to brown, about 10 minutes.

Deglaze the pan with the Marsala, if using, and add the broth and the remaining ½ teaspoon salt. Reduce the heat to low to maintain a gentle simmer. Cover and cook for 5 minutes. Uncover the pan, increase the heat to medium, and cook until the liquid has reduced by half, about 5 minutes more. Discard the thyme sprigs, stir in the butter, and serve.

PEAS WITH
BABY LETTUCES

SERVES 4 TO 6

You may have noticed that I don't think of lettuces exclusively as raw vegetables to be eaten in a salad or as a burger topping. Here soft lettuces are briefly braised in a buttery broth for a pretty and delicate spring-like side. They would be equally nice paired with sugar snap peas, asparagus, even quartered radishes—anything light and bright that won't overwhelm the mild lettuces.

1 (10-ounce) bag frozen peas

½ cup vegetable broth, homemade (page 95) or store-bought

½ teaspoon kosher salt, plus more to taste

2 tablespoons unsalted butter

1 tablespoon chopped fresh tarragon

1 cup baby lettuce leaves, such as Little Gem, baby romaine, baby frisée, or mizuna

½ teaspoon fresh lemon juice (optional)

In a medium skillet, combine the peas, broth, and salt. Bring to a boil over high heat. Reduce to medium-high and cook for 2 minutes, or until the peas are bright green and plump. Using the back of a fork, mash the peas slightly, popping about half of them.

Remove the pan from the heat and add the butter and tarragon. Stir to combine, emulsifying the butter and broth. Add the lettuces to the pan and toss just to warm through; season with more salt if needed. Finish with the lemon juice, if desired.

ROASTED CAULIFLOWER WITH GRAPES *and* PISTACHIOS

SERVES 4

The grapes and pistachios are my favorite part of this dish. Roasting concentrates the sweetness of the grapes so they provide a decadent little pop of flavor in every mouthful.

1 medium head of cauliflower, cut into 2-inch florets

3 tablespoons olive oil

1½ teaspoons kosher salt

1 teaspoon ground fennel seeds

1 cup green grapes, halved

⅓ cup pistachios, finely chopped

Preheat the oven to 450°F.

Place the cauliflower on a rimmed baking sheet and toss well with 2 tablespoons of the oil, the salt, and fennel seeds, coating the florets evenly. Roast for 25 minutes, or until the cauliflower is almost tender and beginning to brown. Add the grapes to the baking sheet and toss well to coat with the hot oil. Return to the oven and roast for an additional 10 minutes, or until the cauliflower is golden brown and the grapes are beginning to burst.

Transfer the cauliflower and grapes to a serving bowl and sprinkle with the chopped pistachios. Drizzle with the remaining tablespoon of oil. Serve warm or at room temperature.

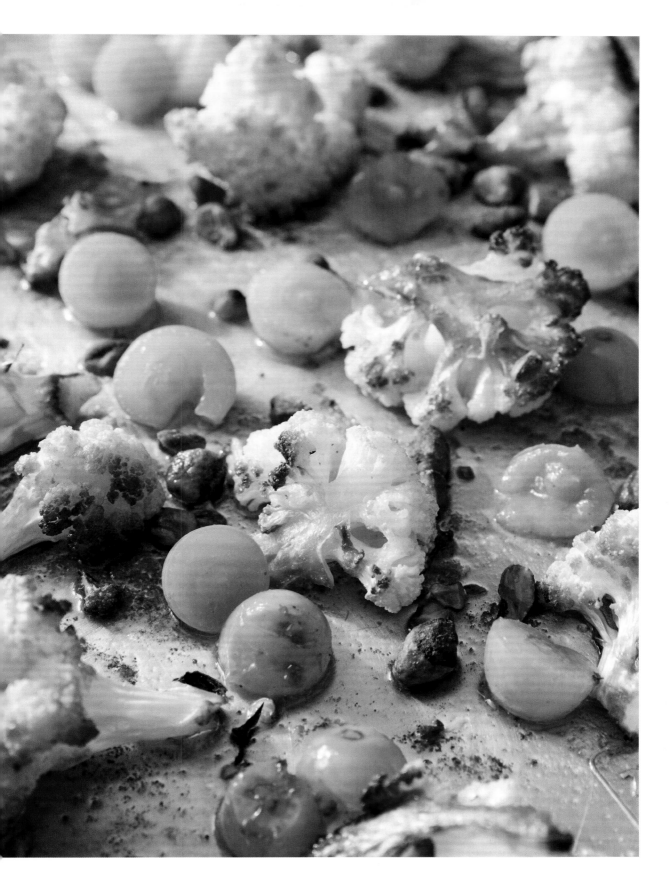

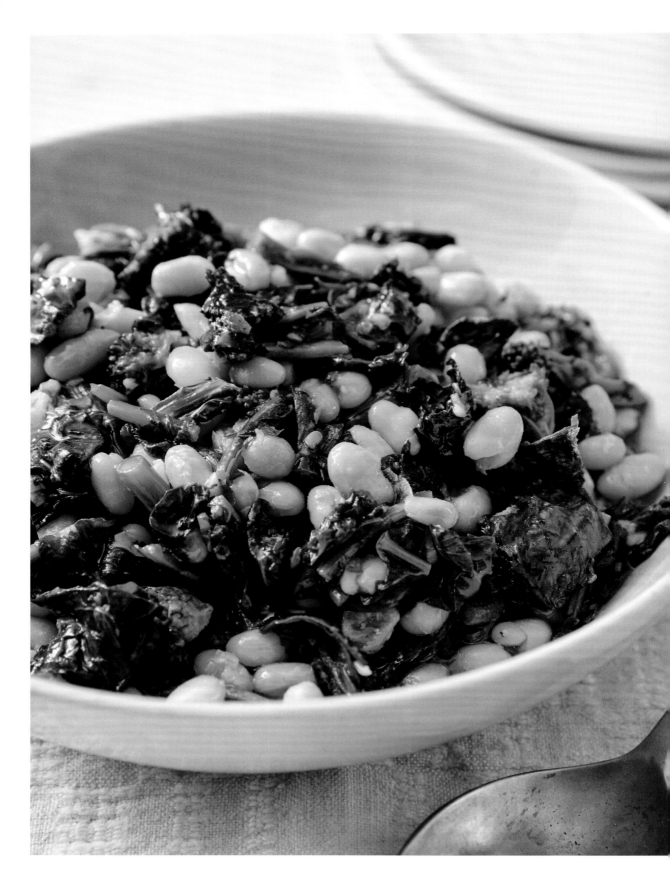

(RB)

WHITE BEAN
and BROCCOLI RABE SAUTÉ

SERVES 4 TO 6

If you've been keeping up with your batch cooking, you may already have cooked beans and broccoli rabe in the fridge, in which case this can be ready in a matter of minutes. Pair this side with a nice piece of broiled fish for a simple but sophisticated meal.

3 tablespoons olive oil, plus more to drizzle

1 bunch of broccoli rabe, trimmed and chopped into 1-inch pieces

½ teaspoon kosher salt

2 cups cooked white or cranberry beans, homemade (page 90) or canned

⅓ cup cooking liquid from the beans, water, or vegetable broth (see Note)

Crushed red pepper flakes (optional)

Heat a large skillet over medium-high heat. Add the olive oil and heat for another minute. Add the broccoli rabe and salt and cook until wilted, about 5 minutes, stirring often. Add the prepared beans with their liquid to the skillet. Simmer for 5 minutes to marry the flavors. Serve drizzled with more olive oil and a sprinkling of red pepper flakes, if using.

NOTE ————

If using canned beans, drain and rinse them well and add about ⅓ cup water or vegetable broth to the pan with the beans.

CURRY-ROASTED BUTTERNUT SQUASH

SERVES 4 TO 6

Almost all hard winter squashes pair beautifully with pumpkin pie spices like cinnamon and cloves. Even without sugar, the combination is just so aromatic and comforting. Curry powder, which contains turmeric and cumin, takes this in an even more savory direction. It's perfect for a fall meal.

1 butternut squash (about 2 pounds), halved lengthwise, seeds discarded

1½ teaspoons kosher salt

4 tablespoons (½ stick) unsalted butter, preferably European-style

½ teaspoon curry powder

Pinch of pumpkin pie spice or a grating of nutmeg

2 tablespoons unsweetened coconut chips

3 tablespoons torn fresh basil leaves

Preheat the oven to 425°F.

Use the tip of a sharp knife to score the cut side of each squash half in a diamond pattern. Season with ½ teaspoon of the salt and set aside.

In a small saucepan, melt the butter with the remaining 1 teaspoon salt, the curry powder, and pumpkin pie spice. Brush the mixture over the scored flesh of the squash.

Roast the squash halves cut side up for 55 minutes, or until the tip of a knife can pierce the flesh with no resistance, basting with more of the butter mixture after about 30 minutes.

To serve, cut each squash half crosswise into 2 or 3 pieces, place on a large platter, and spoon the remaining butter mixture on top. Sprinkle with the coconut and basil. Serve warm.

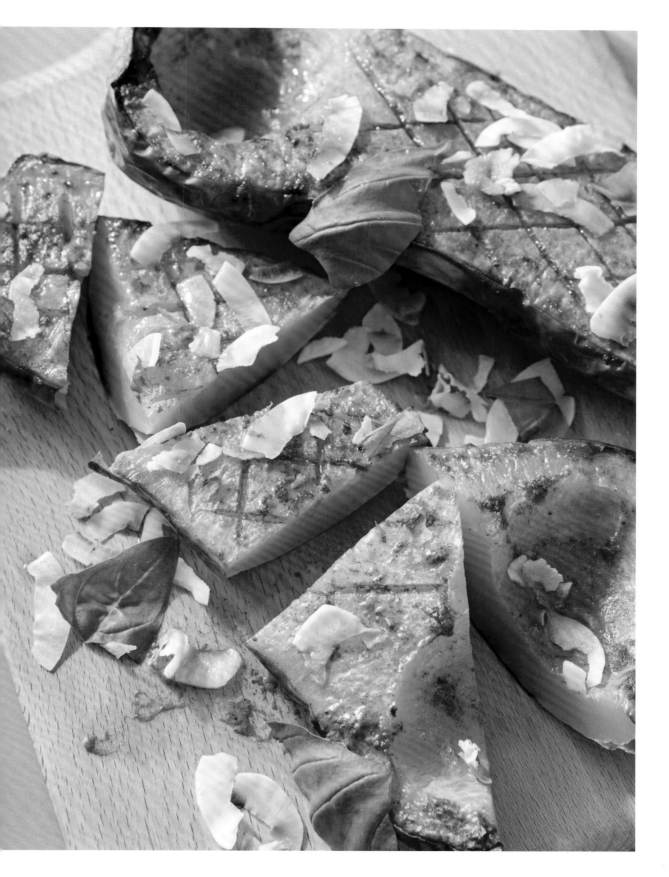

FENNEL-ROASTED YUKON GOLDS

SERVES 4

This recipe gives the people what they want—indulgent, golden roasted potatoes—while stretching the spuds a bit with a less starchy vegetable. Fennel becomes nicely caramelized and sweet when roasted. I think the two textures and flavors work really well together.

2 large Yukon Gold potatoes (about 1 pound), cut into ¼-inch rounds

2 tablespoons olive oil

1 teaspoon kosher salt

1 fennel bulb, stalks removed, sliced into ⅛-inch-thick rings

Preheat the oven to 450°F. Place a rimmed baking sheet in the oven while it heats.

In a medium bowl, toss together the potatoes, olive oil, and ¾ teaspoon of the salt. Using an oven mitt, remove the hot baking sheet from the oven and arrange the potatoes in a single layer, leaving the excess oil in the bowl. Roast the potatoes for 15 minutes.

Meanwhile, add the sliced fennel to the same bowl and sprinkle with the remaining ¼ teaspoon salt. Toss well to coat the fennel in the salt and oil. Remove the potatoes from the oven and turn the slices browned side up. Sprinkle the fennel on top and roast for an additional 20 minutes, or until the potatoes are golden brown and both veggies are tender all the way through.

CAULIFLOWER–SWEET POTATO MASH

SERVES 6

If you are staying away from white potatoes, you should get to know Japanese sweet potatoes. They have off-white flesh and a drier texture than most domestic varieties, and the flavor is more nutty than sweet. Mashing the potato with cauliflower makes for a nice neutral side dish to pair with roasts or chops.

1 large Korean or Japanese sweet potato (about 1 pound), peeled and cut into 2-inch pieces

1 garlic clove, smashed and peeled

1 tablespoon plus 2 teaspoons kosher salt

1 head of cauliflower (about 2 pounds), cut into 2-inch florets

½ cup olive oil

⅛ teaspoon freshly ground black pepper

Place the sweet potato and garlic in a large saucepan with cold water to cover by 3 inches. Bring to a boil over medium-high heat. Season with 1 tablespoon salt and add the cauliflower. Bring back to a boil, then reduce the heat and simmer for about 15 minutes, or until the vegetables are tender when pierced with the tip of a knife. Reserve 3 tablespoons of the cooking liquid, then drain the veggies well.

Working in batches if needed, puree the vegetables in a food processor, adding the remaining 2 teaspoons salt, the olive oil, and the reserved liquid as needed. Transfer the puree to a serving bowl and serve topped with the pepper.

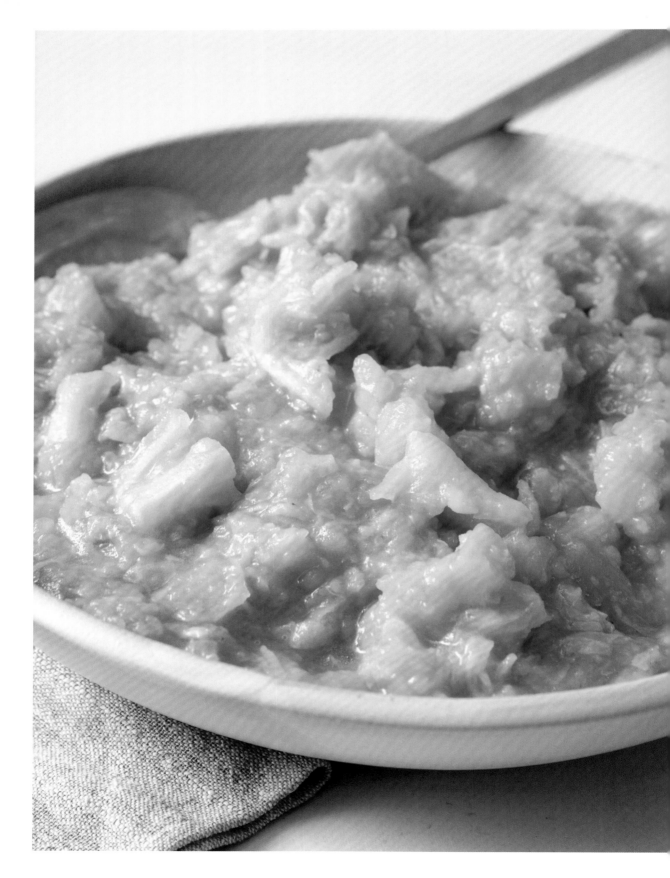

MASHED YUKON GOLDS
WITH SAVOY CABBAGE

SERVES 6

A half cup of oil may sound like a lot, but it gives this mash a velvety texture that's worth the splurge. This dish is on the heavier side, so pair it with something light, like grilled or broiled fish.

½ cup olive oil

1 medium onion, chopped

1 garlic clove, smashed and peeled

2 teaspoons kosher salt

1 small head of savoy cabbage, cut into 1-inch pieces

1 pound Yukon Gold potatoes, peeled and quartered

3½ to 4 cups chicken broth, homemade (page 96) or low-sodium store-bought

Heat a medium Dutch oven over medium heat. Add ¼ cup of the olive oil and the onion and garlic. Season with ½ teaspoon of the salt. Reduce the heat to medium-low and cook the onion slowly, stirring often with a wooden spoon, until soft and tender, about 8 minutes. Add the chopped cabbage and an additional ½ teaspoon of the salt and stir to combine. Cook for 2 minutes, or until the cabbage wilts.

Stir in the potatoes and enough broth to cover the mixture. Season with the remaining teaspoon of salt. Bring the mixture to a simmer and cook, stirring often, until the liquid is reduced by half, the potatoes are tender, and the cabbage is silky and soft, 30 to 35 minutes. Using a potato masher or a whisk, crush the mixture until it loosely resembles the consistency of mashed potatoes. Stir in the remaining ¼ cup olive oil and serve.

CHAPTER 15

Worth It!

Not too many people can go very long without dessert, least of all me. At the end of the day—and that's generally when I start itching for something sugary—life's too short to live without sweets! These days, though, I want to make sure any indulgence is really worth the number I know it may do on my digestion and won't just throw fuel on the fire of my out-of-control sweet tooth.

To make treats that are easier to digest and gentler on my body, I've been experimenting with ingredients I haven't used much before, like alternative flours and sweeteners. Whenever possible I now avoid gluten and highly refined products in my baking and aim to make things just a *little* less sweet than I might have in the past. I find I don't get the same kind of sugar hangover from these desserts, and I enjoy them every bit as much. Before you make these recipes you may need to do a little bit of shopping in the natural products aisle (see page 36 for my list of baking staples). You'll see, for example, that many of these recipes call for coconut sugar rather than regular granulated sugar. I've switched because coconut sugar is less processed than cane sugar and has a slight molasses flavor that I really enjoy. If it's not your cup of tea, though, just swap in the same amount of regular sugar—I'd recommend one of the organic cane sugars that are now widely available. Ultimately, it's all sugar, to be eaten in moderation and mindfully, but you should also enjoy every bite!

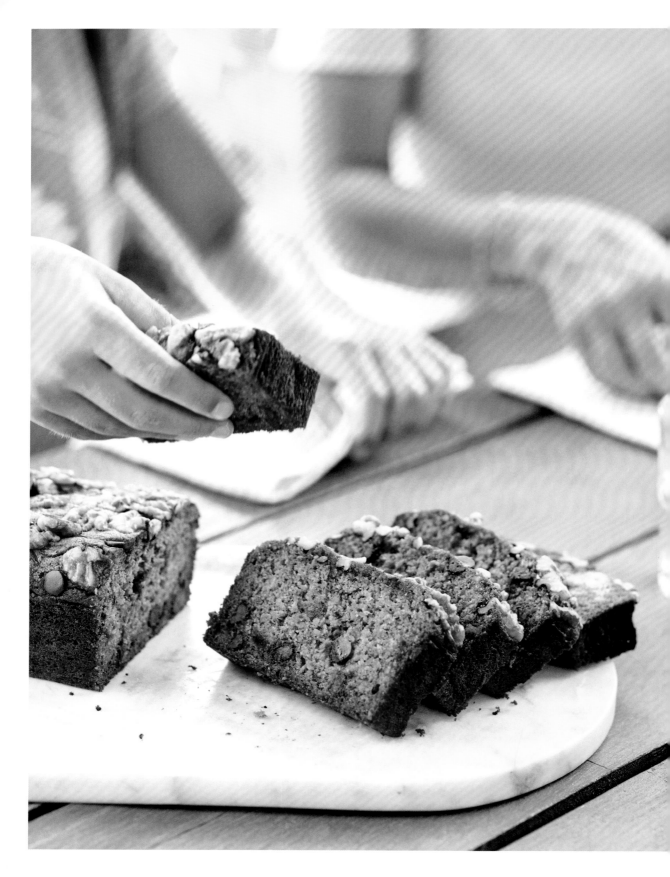

BANANA CHOCOLATE WALNUT BREAD

SERVES 8 TO 10

A combination of chopped walnuts, almond butter, and almond flour gives this loaf a deep, rich flavor that's more sophisticated than your everyday banana bread. The texture is extremely moist even though the recipe doesn't call for much oil. You don't even need a mixer to make it—it's all done in one bowl with a fork and a spatula. Don't underbake this bread; it will get very dark but don't worry, it's not burned! I make this in an oversize loaf pan; if you only have a standard 9 × 5-inch pan, scoop out a half cup or so to cook as a muffin or mini loaf.

3 tablespoons coconut oil, melted and cooled, plus more for the pan

3 very ripe bananas

1 large egg

⅓ cup smooth roasted almond butter

¾ cup organic cane sugar

½ teaspoon kosher salt

¾ cup unsweetened almond milk, homemade (page 104), or store-bought

1 teaspoon pure vanilla extract

1 cup almond flour

1 cup rice flour

2 teaspoons baking soda

½ teaspoon ground cinnamon

½ cup bittersweet chocolate chips, such as Guittard extra-dark (optional)

½ cup chopped walnuts

Preheat the oven to 350°F. Lightly brush the inside of a 10 × 5-inch loaf pan with coconut oil and place a long strip of parchment paper in the bottom, allowing the excess to go up and over each end of the pan. Set aside.

In a large bowl, mash the bananas with the back of a fork until only a few lumps remain. Add the egg and mix with the fork until smooth. Stir in the almond butter, coconut oil, sugar, salt, almond milk, and vanilla and mix with the fork until smooth and incorporated. Add the almond flour, rice flour, baking soda, and cinnamon. Use a rubber spatula to stir until combined. Stir in the chocolate chips, if using.

Pour the batter into the prepared pan and smooth the top. Sprinkle with the walnuts. Bake for 65 to 75 minutes, or until the bread is firm to the touch and a toothpick inserted in the center comes out with very few crumbs. Allow to cool for 30 minutes in the pan with the pan resting on its side. Loosen the edges with a knife and transfer to a wire rack to cool completely. The bread will keep for 4 days at room temperature or can be sliced and frozen for up to a month.

SPICED APPLE MUFFINS

MAKES 12 MUFFINS

Muffins get a bad rap as an excuse for eating cake for breakfast, but as a dessert, or even an afternoon snack, these have a lot going for them—they are tender, moist, and not too sweet. I make them as a healthy-ish snack for Jade, especially in the fall; I love the way the smell of apples and cinnamon baking fills the house.

6 tablespoons (¾ stick) unsalted butter, preferably European-style, at room temperature

⅔ cup coconut sugar

2 large eggs, at room temperature

1 cup rice flour

1 cup almond flour

½ teaspoon baking powder

½ teaspoon baking soda

¼ teaspoon kosher salt

1 teaspoon ground cinnamon

½ cup low-fat plain Greek yogurt, at room temperature

1 medium Granny Smith apple, peeled and cut into ¼-inch dice

⅓ cup sliced almonds

Preheat the oven to 350°F. Grease the cups of a standard 12-cup muffin tin with coconut oil or butter or insert paper liners in the cups.

In a large bowl, beat the butter and sugar with a handheld mixer on medium-high speed until light and fluffy, about 3 minutes. Beat in the eggs one at a time. When fully combined, add the rice flour, almond flour, baking powder, baking soda, salt, cinnamon, yogurt, and ¼ cup water. Beat on low speed until only a few streaks remain. Using a rubber spatula, fold in the apple just until fully combined. Do not overmix.

Divide the batter evenly among the muffin cups. Top with the almonds. Bake for 25 to 30 minutes, rotating the muffin tin halfway through, until a toothpick inserted in the middle of a muffin comes out clean. Allow the muffins to cool completely in the pan.

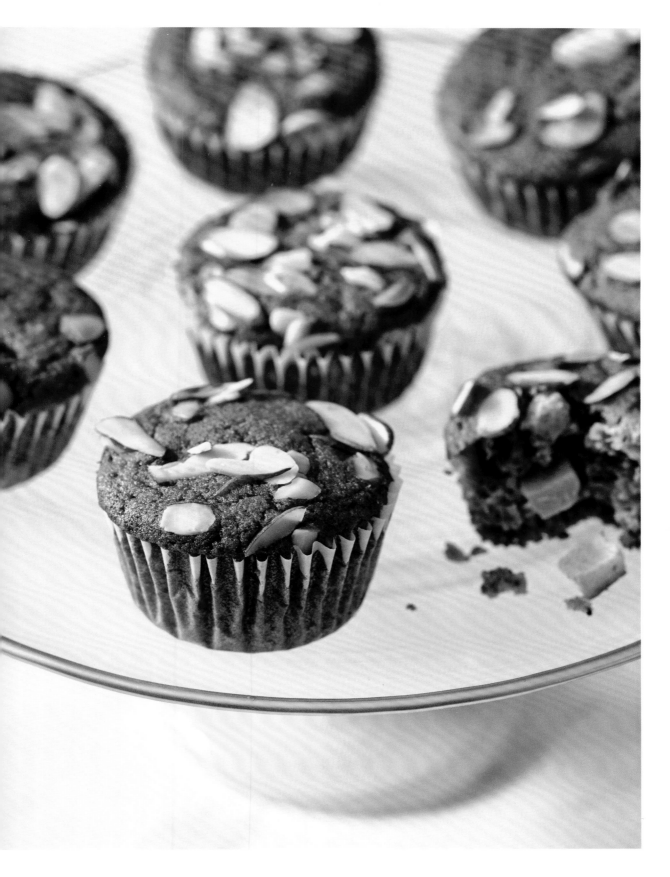

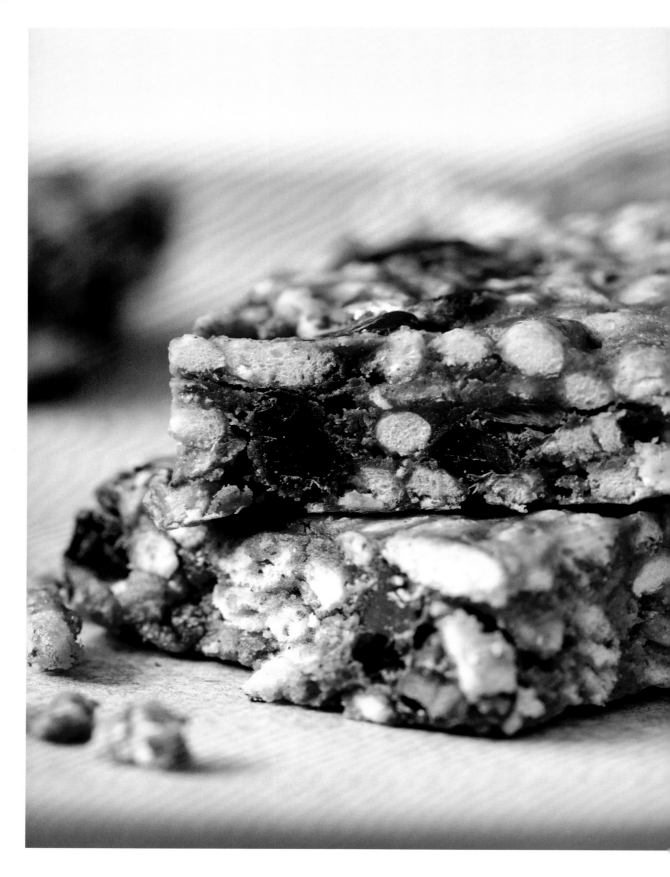

CHOCOLATE *and* ORANGE BROWN RICE TREATS

Crispy rice treats are a guilty pleasure most of us remember from childhood; by swapping out the sugary marshmallow fluff for a caramelly blend of maple syrup and almond butter and adding some grated orange zest, I've transformed them into a sophisticated treat even an adult can love. The nut butter even provides a bit of protein, making them far healthier than the original. The zest gives them a slight bitter edge that I think plays nicely off the chocolate, but Jade doesn't love it, so when I make these for her, I just leave it out. Either way, be sure to let them set for at *least* an hour so they will be firm enough to cut.

Coconut oil, for the pan

3 cups puffed brown rice cereal

½ cup pure maple syrup

⅔ cup creamy almond butter

¼ teaspoon kosher salt

1 teaspoon grated orange zest

½ cup bittersweet chocolate chips, such as Guittard extra-dark

Lightly grease an 8-inch square baking dish with coconut oil. Line the pan with one strip of parchment paper, overhanging the pan at each end, and set aside.

Place the cereal in a large bowl. In a small saucepan, bring the maple syrup to a simmer over medium heat. Whisk in the almond butter, salt, and orange zest, stirring until smooth. Remove from the heat and pour the mixture over the cereal. Using a rubber spatula, toss to coat well.

When cool to the touch, stir in the chocolate chips. Scrape into the prepared pan and smooth the top. Refrigerate until set, at least 1 hour. Cut into bars and serve.

CHEWY ALMOND *and* CHERRY THUMBPRINT COOKIES

MAKES 24 COOKIES

Cherries and almonds go together like peanut butter and jelly, and that pairing is especially nice in these homey-looking cookies. Toasting the almond flour intensifies the cookies' nutty flavor and makes them extra crisp, so don't skip that step.

4 cups almond flour

⅔ cup coconut sugar

¼ cup honey, such as thyme or clover

¼ teaspoon kosher salt

1 teaspoon grated lemon zest

2 tablespoons limoncello or fresh lemon juice, from 1 lemon

1 large egg

About ¼ cup all-fruit cherry jam

Preheat the oven to 350°F.

Spread the almond flour on a rimmed baking sheet and bake for 10 to 15 minutes, stirring halfway through, until the flour is golden brown and toasted. Immediately scrape it into a medium bowl to cool for 5 minutes. Line the baking sheet with parchment paper and set aside.

To the toasted flour, add the sugar, honey, salt, lemon zest, limoncello, and egg. Using a rubber spatula, stir until well combined.

Scoop the dough onto the prepared baking sheet in heaping tablespoons, leaving 1 inch between cookies. Flatten them slightly with the palm of your hand. Using your thumb, make a small indentation in the center of each cookie. Fill each depression with ½ teaspoon of the cherry jam.

Bake the cookies for 15 to 17 minutes, until golden brown and just set. Allow to cool slightly on the pan for 5 minutes before transferring to a wire rack to cool completely. The cookies can be stored for a day or two in an airtight container or frozen for up to 3 months.

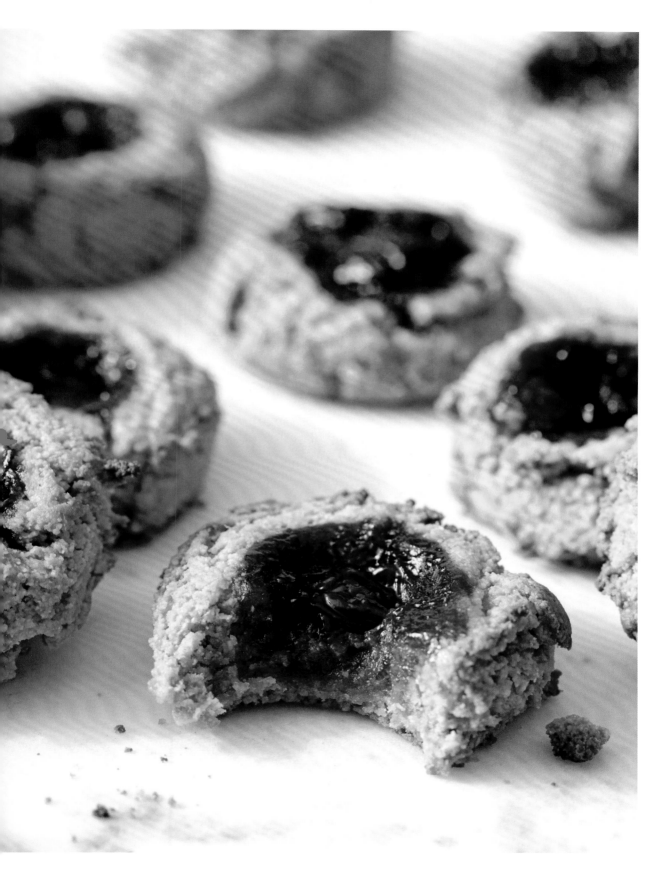

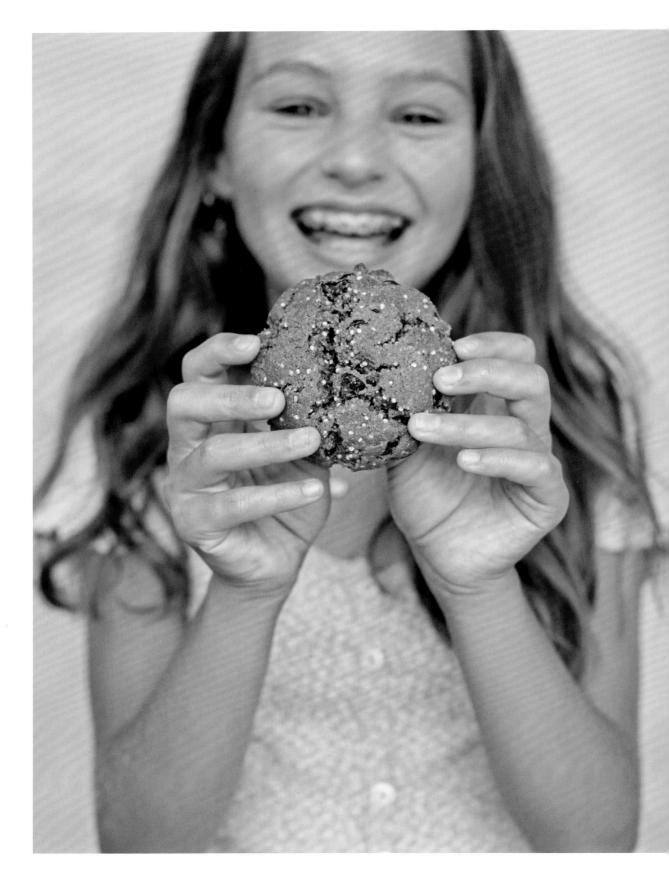

CHOCOLATE CHIP–QUINOA COOKIES

MAKES 12 COOKIES

These have become such a staple in my house that I make them weekly. The toasted quinoa is irresistibly crunchy and, well, chocolate . . . ! Need I say more? They are not at all hard to make, but it is essential that you refrigerate the dough for a good long time—even overnight—or the batter won't be firm enough to scoop and the cookies won't hold their shape as they bake. These are best the day they are made, but they freeze really well (a good way to keep yourself from eating the entire batch at once, btw) and can be eaten straight out of the freezer.

¼ cup quinoa

8 tablespoons (1 stick) unsalted butter, preferably European-style, melted and cooled

1 cup coconut sugar

1 teaspoon pure vanilla extract

1 large egg, at room temperature

1 egg yolk, at room temperature

1 cup almond flour

½ cup coconut flour

½ teaspoon kosher salt

1 teaspoon baking soda

¾ cup bittersweet chocolate chips, such as Guittard extra-dark

Place the quinoa in a small, dry pan over medium heat. Cook, stirring occasionally, until the quinoa is evenly toasted and beginning to pop, 3 to 4 minutes. Spread on a plate to cool completely.

Combine the melted butter, sugar, and vanilla in a mixing bowl and stir to combine. Add the egg and egg yolk and whisk until smooth. Add the almond flour, coconut flour, salt, and baking soda and stir to form a soft dough. Add the toasted quinoa and chocolate chips and stir until evenly distributed. Refrigerate for at least 4 hours and up to 24 hours.

Preheat the oven to 350°F. Line a rimmed baking sheet with parchment paper.

Scoop ¼-cup balls of dough onto the prepared baking sheet, placing them 2 inches apart. Flatten them slightly with the bottom of a glass or the heel of your hand. Bake for 13 to 15 minutes, rotating the pan halfway through, until the edges are just set and the centers are still slightly underdone. Cool on the baking sheet for 10 minutes before transferring to a wire rack to cool completely. Don't store these cookies. Freeze any you haven't eaten within 8 hours; they'll keep for up to a month.

COCONUT
RICE PUDDING

SERVES 4

Rice pudding = comfort food for a lot of people. Made with Arborio rice, this vegan version is every bit as creamy as you'd expect from a classic "nursery" dessert, without all the dairy. The optional toppings add a bit of textural contrast, but either way this is deeply soothing and satisfying.

2 (13.5-ounce) cans light coconut milk

¾ cup Arborio rice, rinsed

¾ teaspoon kosher salt

½ cup coconut sugar

½ teaspoon ground cinnamon

1 teaspoon pure vanilla extract

1 teaspoon grated lemon zest

Unsweetened shaved coconut flakes, bittersweet chocolate chips, or toasted slivered almonds, for garnish (optional)

In a medium saucepan, combine the coconut milk, 2 cups water, the rice, salt, sugar, cinnamon, and vanilla. Bring to a simmer over medium heat, then reduce the heat to medium-low to maintain a gentle simmer. Cook, stirring often with a rubber spatula, for about 20 minutes, or until the rice is just cooked through. Remove from the heat and stir in the lemon zest. Cool for 20 minutes, then transfer to individual serving dishes or a large bowl, cover, and refrigerate for at least 1 hour, or until completely chilled.

Serve topped with coconut, chocolate chips, or slivered almonds, or a combination of the three, if desired.

MIXED BERRIES WITH SPICED MAPLE SYRUP

SERVES 4

When I host dinner parties, I prefer to offer something light at the end of the meal, and this fits the bill perfectly, because it's both elegant and simple to make. It's especially nice in the summer, when there is a lot of fresh fruit around—here I use mixed berries, but you can adapt it to whatever is in season, such as sliced plums or nectarines. You will have more syrup than you need, but the extra is wonderful served over pancakes.

½ cup pure maple syrup

1 cinnamon stick

1 star anise

½ teaspoon whole cloves

Pinch of kosher salt

3 cups mixed berries, rinsed and halved (or quartered if large)

¼ cup plain Greek yogurt (optional)

In a small saucepan, combine the maple syrup, cinnamon, star anise, cloves, and salt. Bring to a simmer over medium heat, then reduce the heat and simmer gently for 5 minutes. Remove from the heat and allow the mixture to cool completely. Strain the syrup through a fine-mesh strainer, discarding the spices.

Divide the berries among four coupes or dessert dishes. Dollop with the yogurt, if using, and drizzle each serving with 1 to 2 teaspoons of the syrup. Leftover syrup will keep for up to 2 weeks in a sealed jar in the refrigerator.

NO-COOK CHOCOLATE COCONUT BUDINO

SERVES 6

Budino is Italian for "pudding," and I've loved budinos of all kinds since I was a kid. Now that I'm an adult, though, I find the dairy in a typical pudding or custard just kills me. So when I need something smooth, creamy, and decadent, I make this vegan budino that's not too sweet, and it's all good.

¼ cup good-quality unsweetened cocoa powder

3 tablespoons pure maple syrup

1 teaspoon pure vanilla extract

Pinch of kosher salt

¾ cup unsweetened almond milk, homemade (page 104), or store-bought

¾ cup coconut yogurt, such as COYO or Anita's

⅓ cup chia seeds

Toasted unsweetened coconut flakes, toasted sliced almonds, or mixed berries, for garnish (optional)

In a medium bowl, whisk together the cocoa, maple syrup, vanilla, salt, almond milk, and yogurt until smooth. Stir in the chia seeds.

Cover and refrigerate for at least 6 hours, or until thickened to the consistency of pudding. Serve topped with toasted coconut flakes, nuts, or berries, if desired.

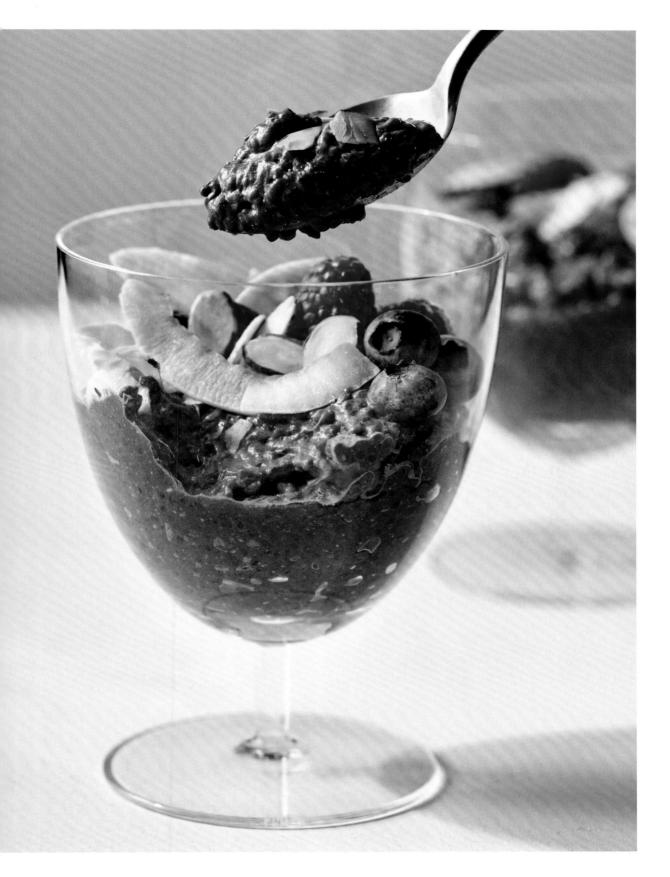

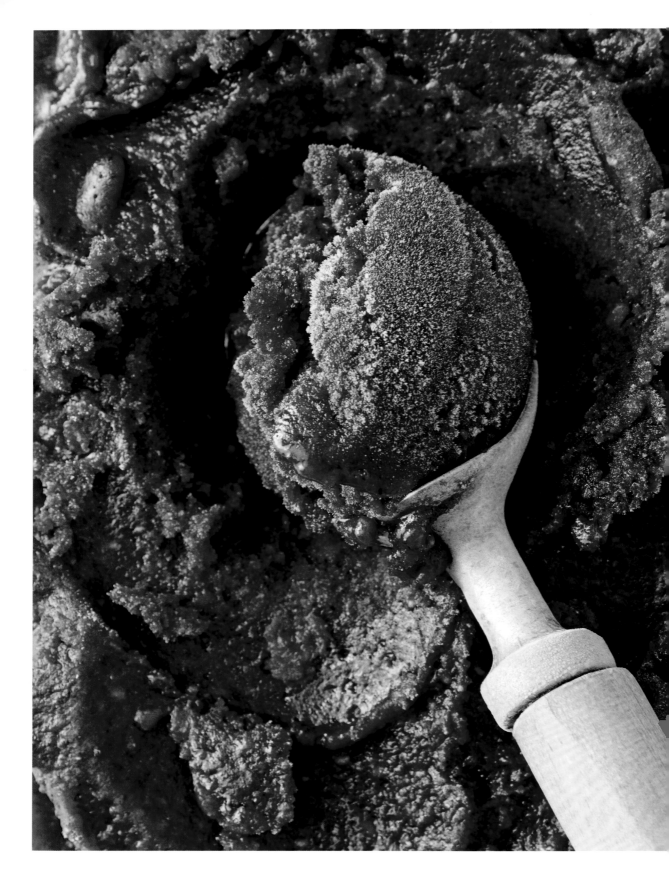

SIMPLE SORBETTO

SERVES 2

Desserts don't get much simpler than this, and the flavor is as bright and vivid as the color. Adding a tablespoon of vodka to the berry mixture keeps the sorbetto from freezing completely, so it's still soft enough to scoop if you make it ahead of time. If you're serving it to kids, leave it out, obviously!

1 (10-ounce) bag frozen mixed berries

¼ cup pure maple syrup

Pinch of salt

1 tablespoon vodka (optional)

Combine the berries, maple syrup, salt, and vodka, if using, in a blender. Pulse the mixture to create a coarse puree. Scrape down the sides of the blender with a rubber spatula. Continue to pulse, scraping down the sides as needed, until smooth and scoopable.

Serve immediately or transfer to an airtight container and freeze for up to a week.

ROASTED STRAWBERRIES WITH VIN SANTO

SERVES 4

If you like strawberries with balsamic, give this more subtle cooked version a try. It's everything I look for in a dessert: fast, easy, and impressive. People ooh and aah every time I serve it, and it's easy to multiply for a crowd.

1 pound strawberries, hulled and halved

1 tablespoon plus 1 teaspoon coconut sugar or organic cane sugar

2 teaspoons olive oil

Pinch of kosher salt

¼ cup Vin Santo or other dessert wine (optional)

½ cup coconut yogurt, such as COYO or Anita's

¼ cup coarsely chopped Marcona almonds

Preheat the oven to 350°F. Lined a rimmed baking sheet with parchment paper.

Combine the strawberries, 1 tablespoon of the sugar, the olive oil, and salt on the prepared baking sheet and toss well to coat. Spread the strawberries evenly and roast for 30 minutes, or until they are soft and have released some of their juices. Pour the berries and their juices into a bowl and gently stir in the Vin Santo, if using. Cool to room temperature.

To serve, whisk the yogurt and the remaining 1 teaspoon sugar together in a small bowl. Divide the berries among four small serving dishes. Dollop the yogurt on top and sprinkle each serving with some of the chopped almonds.

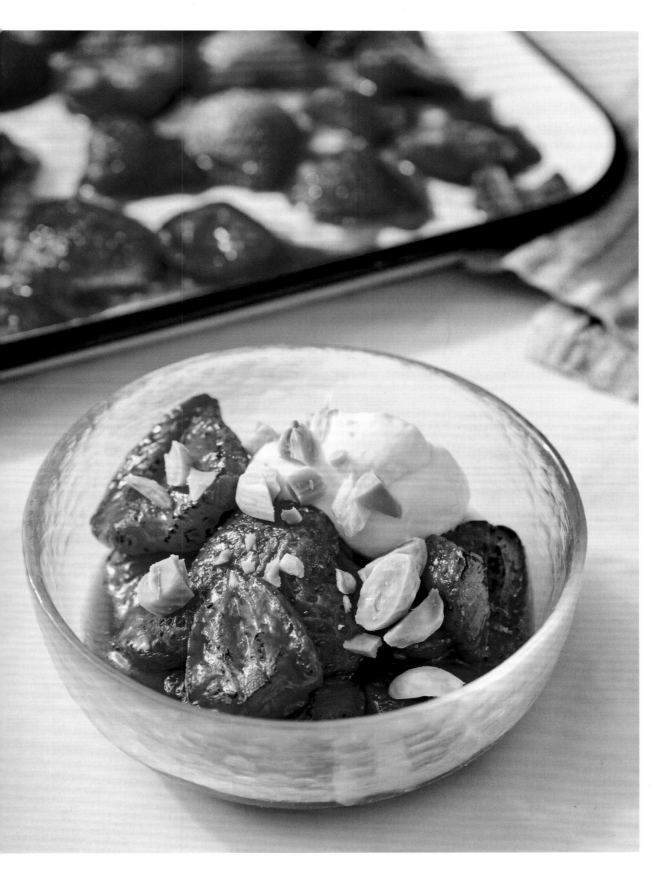

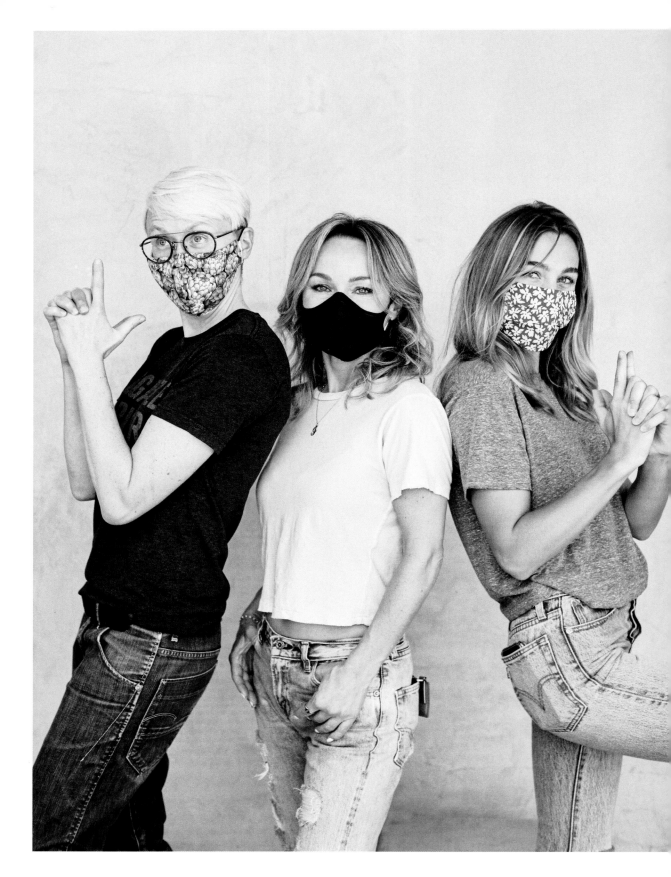

ACKNOWLEDGMENTS

This book is inspired by a journey of health and wellness that enlisted the help of many talented people. I want to thank everyone who contributed to making it a reality.

We shot the photos during one of the biggest health crises in modern history—a very surreal moment. The crew was small, but there were a lot of people on the periphery who helped it come to fruition:

* Kristin, David, and Kate: Thanks for all your patience and for keeping us laughing.

* Lish and Rosecleer: Thanks for keeping the deliciousness coming all day long.

* Janeva Turton: Thank you for your determination to find the right ingredients. They made all the difference.

* Darcy Gilmore and Havana Prats: Like knights in shining armor with masks and shields, you came to rescue me and turn me into a little princess. Thank you!

* Le Creuset and Made In generously supplied products for these photos.

Thanks also to:

* Natasha Wynnyk: Thank you for being my all-in-one, from keeping everyone safe from COVID-19 to being an animal wrangler and the #1 TikTok curator— you were our Swiss army knife!

* Lindsey Galey and Lizzy Newman: Thanks for your digital support from afar.

* Jade Thompson and Shane Farley: Thanks for being my #1 taste testers.

* Pam Krauss: You have a way with words that I admire and aspire to every day. Thank you for helping me get my thoughts together in a way that actually makes sense!

* Everyone at Crown Publishing/ Rodale, including, Gina Centrello, Aaron Wehner, Diana Baroni, Raquel Pelzel, Marysarah Quinn, Mia Johnson, Christina Foxley, Tammy Blake, Emily Isayeff, Leilani Zee, and Emily Hotaling.

* Dr. Deborah Kim: Thank you for guiding me through this process and for responding to my random text messages with crazy medical questions at all hours. You inspire me to stay on top of my health and wellness every day.

* Eric Greenspan, Suzanne Gluck, and Jon Rosen: Thank you for your continued dedication and support.

And always a special thanks to my family—because without their support, I wouldn't be where I am today.

Lastly, a special thanks to my animal family: Bella, Bruno, and Luna, who generously gave their time for the photos.

Note: Page references
in *italics* indicate
photographs.

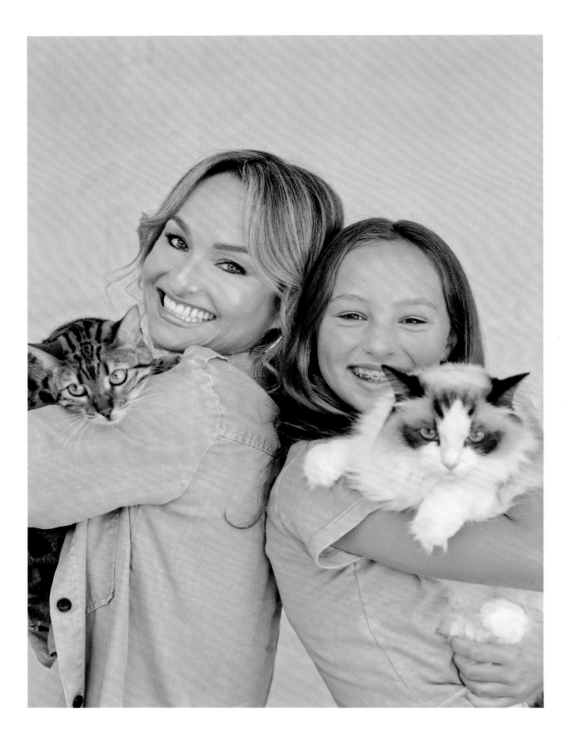